FERT

JULIE REID is a naturopath, medical herbalist and acupuncturist who has been in clinical practice for 24 years. She has written for the media on health and nutrition and lectured internationally to health professionals, students and lay people.

Overcoming Common Problems Series

For a full list of titles please contact
Sheldon Press, Marylebone Road, London NW1 4DU

Overcoming Common Problems Series

Overcoming Common Problems Series

Overcoming Common Problems

Fertility
A natural approach

Julie Reid

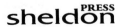
sheldon PRESS

First published in Great Britain in 2001
Sheldon Press
Holy Trinity Church
Marylebone Road
London NW1 4DU

First published in New Zealand in 1999 by Tandem Press

British Library Cataloguing in Publication Data
A catalogue record for this book is available from the British Library

ISBN 0–85969–855–6

Typeset by Deltatype Limited, Birkenhead, Merseyside
Printed in Great Britain by
Biddles Ltd., Guildford and King's Lynn

Contents

Preface

Thank heavens this book is available. It could have saved us ten frustrating, stressful, roller-coaster years. We were both 30 when we returned home from an overseas stay. Income was secure, we had a house with a garden, a cat, goldfish, and finches followed. The stage for a family was set. We were just waiting for the appearance of the elusive central characters. Then the emotional ups and downs began. Hopes rose and fell with each monthly cycle. Two years on we decided to seek specialist help. If something was wrong, we decided, we should have it fixed so we could get on with having a family.

After several weeks of tests, 'unexplained infertility' was the diagnosis. Mike's sperm count was high but motility was low. A post-coital test showed that my system was killing off most of his sperm. Why? Nobody could tell us. The prognosis was a greatly reduced chance of that desperately desired pregnancy. There were more tears, depression and anger at the unfairness of it all. Why us? It seemed everyone we knew was busy, not on number one but numbers two or three.

One option that could bypass any malfunction in our bodies was GIFT (gamete intra-fallopian transfer). This involved two weeks of fertility drugs to stimulate egg production, followed by daily blood tests to determine hormone readiness levels for egg pick-up via laparoscopy. Scans of ovaries were also carried out to determine the number and size of the collectable eggs. About one day before my eggs would naturally be released from the ovaries, I was given a general anaesthetic to enable laparoscopic egg collection. These eggs were mixed with Mike's sperm and returned to my fallopian tubes hopefully to join forces to create a new life.

Optimism was high for that first attempt. Over three thousand pounds and a few weeks later we were informed that it had not been successful. We braced ourselves for two more tries, with ever-diminishing optimism. The third effort produced brief joy, despite my feeling incredibly sick the whole time. The joy turned to despair and numbness six weeks later when a scan showed the spark of embryonic life was no more.

We would go no further along this path. That was it. We felt emotionally, mentally and physically wrung out. I couldn't face any more needles or medical probing of my body. We did get on with life, but I could not accept our childless condition as final. The biological clock would not be silenced as we headed down the unwelcoming childless path to forty. Our reading and delving began to lead to the common-sense approach of natural remedies such as dietary changes, relaxation, and mineral and vitamin therapy to bring our bodies to a healthier state of balance. Job changes ensued.

One year into Mike's new job with a leading natural healthcare company, and at the end of my first of a four-year naturopathic course, I became pregnant. An interesting coincidence, some may say, but so was listening to inspiring speakers such as Julie Reid and following her dietary, mineral and vitamin guidance. One of the benefits of this nutritional approach was better health and wellbeing. Sinus problems improved, but of course for us the results included a very healthy pregnancy and a beautiful healthy baby boy. What a way to celebrate our fortieth year.

Medically assisted conceptions work for some, but for many others, an awful lot of time, energy, stress and money can be saved by applying natural remedies and the suggestions outlined in this book. We certainly wish we had followed this path earlier to have had the pleasure of our son sooner and at a younger age ourselves.

Read this book. Share it with others. You might be surprised at the number of couples having difficulty conceiving. Trying to have a baby can place individuals and relationships under enormous stress. Friends or family often wish to help but do not know how to without upsetting what is often a sensitive situation. A discreet suggestion to read this book may be the best gift that you could give a couple and that they could receive. If you have been trying for a baby for some time, remember it is always challenging and satisfying to take more control over your own health and fertility. Go for it! You have nothing to lose and heaps to gain.

Our heartfelt best wishes

Vivien and Mike Byrnes

Vivien is a qualified teacher and has trained as a naturopath. Mike is a past president both of the National Nutritional Foods Association (NNFA) and the Non-Prescription Medicines Association (NMA), in New Zealand.

Acknowledgements

My first word of thanks must go to Linda Cassells for her advice and direction, to Lynda Wharton, who felt this was a book that had to be written, and to all those who made the book a reality.

So many other people have helped in different ways, especially my patients who have given me the privilege of working with them and learning with them. Many of them have kept in touch through the years, telling me of their children's successes. In order to respect their privacy, I have changed their names.

My sincerest thanks to Mim Barnes of Foresight who opened all their literature to me so freely, and to John Peek of Fertility Associates who encouraged me to read statistics and other literature related to fertility. To Kathryn Darby of Natural Family Planning, for her advice and encouragement, and to NFP for permission to use their charts in this book. To Neil Ward, Director of Research in the Department of Chemistry, University of Surrey, for his interest in the project.

Thanks also to the following fellow practitioners who contributed so enthusiastically during the preparation of the manuscript and who shared their case histories – Martin Greenleaf (acupuncture); Bruce Barwell (homoeopathy); Dr Jarrod Appleton (osteopathy); Jenny Mitchell (aromatherapy and massage); and Joan Lust (sex therapy).

My thanks to fellow practitioner and friend Carol Mosedale, who so readily helped with research and tracking down lots of little but necessary things, and who with my sister-in-law Linda read and re-read the manuscript.

Thanks also to my teacher and friend Les Fisher who, some 20 years ago, made me realize the importance of deficiencies at cellular level, and through the years has been so generous in sharing his incredible knowledge and expertise.

To my nephew Nick Taylor, who is just embarking on his art career, thank you for the original sketches.

Finally my special thanks to George, who put me and this project before anything else, and to my wonderful sons and daughters-in-law, Duncan, Douglas, Rosalind and Megan, who gave me help in so many ways and were able to keep smiling while trying to make me more computer-literate. That was probably the hardest task of all. Thank you everybody.

Introduction

Back in 1981 my interest in mineral deficiencies and fertility was fired when a patient who was seeking help for her migraines and pre-menstrual problems became pregnant two months after starting her naturopathic treatment. It was only later that she mentioned she had been trying to conceive for 11 years. She and her husband had exhausted all medical help, and rather than continue to hope, they had tried to put the issue behind them. So began an aspect of my work that involved much research, uncovering many interesting studies on the importance of nutrition and fertility.

We hear a lot about high-tech fertility clinics that bring hope to many couples wanting to conceive a baby. The success rate for *in vitro* fertilization (IVF) is cited at 20 per cent per treatment cycle, and 29 per cent for gamete intra-fallopian transfer (GIFT). Yet little is known about the thousands of couples who have followed the natural approach for enhancing their fertility, the success rate of which is, conservatively, 90 per cent for a nutritionally based programme. A study conducted by Surrey University of 367 couples enrolled on a Foresight programme during 1990–2 showed the success rate for healthy full-term babies to previously infertile couples to be 86 per cent. Foresight's overall statistics indicate a 91 per cent success rate of take-home healthy babies.

There is much scientific research showing the benefits of nutritional therapy, herbal medicine and acupuncture, and clinical evidence that some other natural therapies help enhance fertility. When administered by qualified practitioners, they are safe, there are no side effects or emotional trauma, and your overall health is improved. Healthy bodies do make beautiful, healthy babies – with very little trouble at all. This book is not a guide to self-diagnosis. It is intended to help you understand more about subfertility and to encourage a greater awareness of various approaches to restoring the body to its fertile state.

As you read this book, forget about the words 'fault' and 'blame'. Both these words will no doubt have been bandied about in private conversations. In the days and months ahead, remember to love each other well, and learn to work with and trust your bodies. And relax. I have found that if patients work towards maximizing their health and forget about 'trying too hard', conception often results.

Part 1: Fertility Problems – The Facts and Causes

1
Subfertility

Before considering ways in which fertility can be enhanced, it is necessary to understand how pregnancy occurs in the first place. In this section we look at how the male and female reproductive systems work, in well-functioning bodies. We then identify the main causes, physical and otherwise, of problems associated with fertility.

What is Subfertility?

Human reproduction is such a complex, chance procedure, it is a wonder conception occurs as frequently and in some cases as easily as it does. A healthy man is constantly fertile, but females are only fertile for a few days every month. Even if intercourse takes place over the mid-cycle fertile days, there is only a 20 per cent chance for young couples that conception will take place, and that chance diminishes with each passing year after the age of 30. This is how it has to be in the broader scheme of things, otherwise population explosions would be rife. In effect, we are a subfertile species.

For a couple having problems producing just one child, this is no doubt the last thing you want to hear. However, the following figures may give you some solace:

- The average time it takes for a pregnancy to occur is between four and six months.
- Eighty per cent of couples conceive within 18 months of trying for a pregnancy.
- Ninety per cent of couples conceive after trying for two years.

This means very few couples are actually infertile. *Subfertile*, yes, but not infertile. There is a difference.

Subfertility and Infertility – What's the Difference?

Subfertility is reduced or impaired fertility, including miscarriage. It is also unexplained infertility, which means that no medical cause can be found for the problem.

Infertility or sterility, on the other hand, involves physiological abnormalities that make it impossible to conceive or hold a pregnancy.

In males the causes of infertility are:

- an absence of sperm (azoospermia);
- congenital defects;
- blockages of the epididymis or vas deferens;
- testicle damage;
- retrograde ejaculation;
- impotence.

The causes of infertility in females are:

- blockages of, or absence of, fallopian tube;
- absence or abnormality of reproductive organs;
- absence of ovulation (anovulation).

In both the male and the female sexually transmitted diseases such as chlamydia and gonorrhoea can cause infertility.

With the advances in microsurgery and assisted conception, some of the conditions listed above can now be overcome. So even for an infertile couple, high technology and the skill of the fertility experts can bring about a miracle. What is seldom considered is that the success of such procedures would be greatly enhanced, and the resulting baby stronger and healthier, if a simple nutritional regime were followed prior to and during the treatment and pregnancy.

You are generally diagnosed as being 'infertile' if you have been having unprotected sex at frequent intervals (two or three times a week) for a period of 12 months with no pregnancy resulting. Some researchers think that help should be sought after eight months of trying to conceive. Others say the timeframe for diagnosis should be two years, but realize that many couples will wish to do something about becoming pregnant long before 24 cycles have passed.

Who Suffers from Subfertility?

UK figures during the 1980s showed that 10–15 per cent of couples were affected by fertility problems. One in five pregnancies resulted in a miscarriage, and one in 16 in a malformed baby. Today statistics tell us that some 25 per cent of couples will have difficulty conceiving at some time during their reproductive life.

So you are certainly not alone – although you will often feel as if you are the only couple in the world not able to produce a baby. It is important to remember that subfertility is not a permanent condition. But before looking at ways of enhancing fertility, it is essential to understand what happens when our reproductive system is working as it should – perfectly.

2

Understanding Our Bodies

Our Hormones

Hormones are the controlling factors of the male and female reproductive systems, so they are a good place to begin. Hormones are produced by tiny glands in the brain and endocrine system, and together with the nervous system regulate our metabolism. They are chemical compounds or 'messengers' that circulate in the blood and influence tissues in other parts of the body to behave in a specific way. The hormones that control both the male and female reproductive systems are released mainly from the brain and the pituitary gland. The two main hormones are the follicle stimulating hormone (FSH) and the luteinizing hormone (LH). In the male FSH and LH influence the testes and the production of sperm. In the female the two hormones regulate the menstrual cycle, and bring about changes in the uterus and cervix.

The Male Factor

Everything begins with the sperm, millions of which are produced constantly. They begin their life in the *testes*, which are encased within the *scrotum*, the pouch-like structure behind the *penis*. The testes contain about 75 cm of *seminiferous tubules*. Here the sperm are produced by a process known as 'spermatogenesis', which takes 48 days.

The sperm pass through this extended network of tubules, which ultimately carries them through the capsule of the testes into the *epididymis*, a convoluted duct about 6 metres in length that lies above and behind the testes, where they spend approximately 14 days. They then pass into a larger tube, the *vas deferens*. While the sperm are being moved through these tubes, they go through a maturing process, aided by secretions from the *seminal vesicle*, a small sac at the base of the *vas deferens* and the *prostate gland*, which is about the size of a walnut and surrounds the neck of the bladder. These secretions protect, nourish and transport sperm, promoting fertility and fertilization. The sperm are held in the vas

Figure 1 Male sex organs

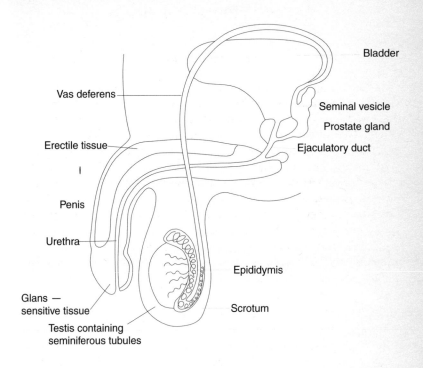

deferens until they pass into the urethra to be released from the *glans* of the penis during ejaculation.

Until the sperm are released from the penis high into the female vagina, each one is coated with a protein substance which renders them 'sleepy'. The sperms' real energy must be conserved for that final 'dash' to meet the egg at the very end of its journey, deep within the female pelvis.

The Female Body

The external female genitals are collectively known as the *vulva*. It includes the *mons pubis*, a fatty pad which is covered in pubic hair, the *labia majora* (outer lips) and *labia minora* (inner lips), which protect the opening of the *vagina*, the *urethral orifice* and the *clitoris*. The clitoris is a knob of erectile tissue rich in nerve ends that lies beneath the hood of skin at the junction of the labia minora. This organ is extremely sensitive and produces intense sexual excitement when stimulated. The *perineum* is the muscular area separating the vagina and *anus*. The *Bartholin's glands*, which lubricate the vagina, are two small rounded bodies on either side of the vaginal opening near the perineum.

The vagina is a hollow muscular tube about 10 cm long, leading from the vulva externally to the uterus, with an amazing ability to expand and contract. At the upper end of the vagina is the *cervix* – the neck of the *uterus*, the small opening of which is called the *os*. This is the passage through which the menstrual blood flows and by which the sperm enter the uterus. The shape and firmness of the cervix changes throughout the menstrual cycle.

The uterus is a hollow organ about the size and shape of an upsidedown pear. It has a blood-rich lining called *endometrium*. This builds up throughout the month and is shed during the menstrual period. On either side of the upper part of the uterus are the *fallopian tubes*, which are about 10 cm long and extend up into the abdomen.

Figure 2 External female genitals

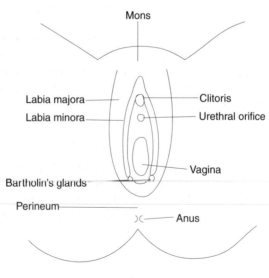

Figure 3 Internal female sex organs

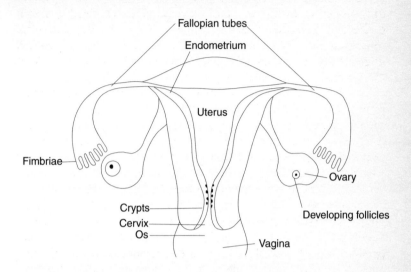

They transport the eggs from the ovaries to the uterus. The outer ends of each fallopian tube are fringed by finger-like projections of tissue called *fimbriae*. It is these 'fingers' that pick up the released egg from the surface of the *ovaries* for transportation through the tube. The almond-shaped ovaries store tiny single-celled eggs that are released each month at ovulation.

A baby girl is born with about a million egg *follicles* (tiny sacs each containing an egg) in her undeveloped ovaries. Throughout her life until menopause the follicles constantly reduce in number, and only about 350 will ever come to full maturity, one each month throughout her reproductive life.

The Menstrual Cycle

The female body is rather like a well-tuned clock, each cycle repeating itself month after month throughout the reproductive years. The menstrual cycle is divided into four phases. A 28-day cycle would look a little like this, give or take a day or two:

A TYPICAL 28-DAY CYCLE	
Stage One	the menstrual period, which lasts about five days
Stage Two	the follicular stage – also known as the post-menstrual, pre-ovulatory, or proliferative phase (owing to the effect of oestrogen on the endometrium), which lasts about nine days
Stage Three	ovulation, which occurs on day 15 or 16
Stage Four	the luteal phase – also known as the post-ovulatory or pre-menstrual phase. This is the progesterone phase, which lasts 12–16 days

The first day of the menstrual bleed is day one of the cycle. Bleeding typically lasts five days. Once the menstrual cycle begins, the brain releases a hormone called gonadotropin, which signals the pituitary gland to release the follicle stimulating hormone (FSH), which in turn signals the ovaries to begin ripening the follicles. (About 20 follicles per cycle are ripened during the prime reproductive years, but the number diminishes with age.) As the follicles mature over the next 14 days they produce an increasing amount of oestrogen which is released into the blood. Oestrogen has many effects on the body, and at this stage of the cycle it renders the cervical mucus fertile, softens and widens the os, thickens the endometrium, and sends signals back to the pituitary gland to reduce the FSH output. This pre-ovulatory part of the cycle is known as the proliferative or follicular phase.

There will only be sufficient FSH in the blood to ripen one, the strongest, follicle. The others disintegrate. The strong maturing follicle pours oestrogen into the body, which has the further effect of diminishing the output of FSH, and triggering the release of the luteinizing hormone (LH). Two to three days later the egg pops from the follicle. Ovulation has taken place. It is generally thought that women ovulate in the late afternoon, so intercourse in the morning (when testosterone is high and your partner eager) will get the sperm in the right place at the right time.

Once ovulation has occurred, the second half of the cycle begins. This is known as the luteal, post-ovulatory or pre-menstrual phase,

Figure 4 The four stages of the menstrual cycle

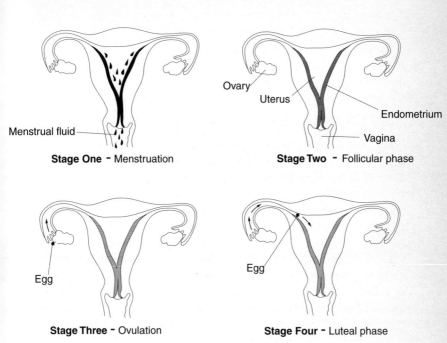

Stage One - Menstruation

Stage Two - Follicular phase

Stage Three - Ovulation

Stage Four - Luteal phase

and is dominated by progesterone. The empty follicle is now known as the *corpus luteum* ('yellow body' referring to the yellowish fat in it). The corpus luteum is a short-lived minute gland that produces progesterone. Progesterone, together with diminishing oestrogen levels, has the effect of further thickening and enriching the endometrium with glands and blood vessels. Should fertilization of the egg take place, conditions will be perfect for receiving and nurturing the fertilized egg. If fertilization does not take place, progesterone levels fall as the corpus luteum disintegrates, and the endometrium, along with blood, is shed as menstruation begins – and with it a new cycle.

It is the follicular phase that is variable in length, giving some women a longer or shorter cycle than the typical 28 days. In a longer cycle, which is more usual than a shorter cycle, of say 32 days, ovulation probably occurs on day 19. The day of ovulation generally occurs on the same day every month for the duration of a woman's reproductive life. It can, however, be delayed by stress, trauma, travel, illness or changes in lifestyle such as excessive exercise or crash diets.

Your monthly cycle should be regular and trouble free. If it is, then this indicates that your hormones are as finely tuned as nature intended. Nobody should suffer from pre-menstrual or menstrual distress. If you do experience problems, they are a reflection of your nutritional status, or indicate a structural problem or an energy imbalance. Most problems of this nature can be simply corrected with a treatment of minerals, with herbs, acupuncture or osteopathy, depending on what the cause is.

Fertilization

Once the egg is picked up from the surface of the ovaries by the fimbriae it may be fertilized in the *ampulla* of the fallopian tubes. If fertilization occurs, the egg will remain here in a nutrient-rich mucus for two to three days. The mucus then becomes less dense and the egg is moved through the microscopic *isthmus* by tiny hairs (*cilia*) of the intricate tube lining. Here the egg (now divided into 16 cells) stays for about 30 hours before arriving in the uterus, and three days later the new embryo is implanted in the lining of the uterus, the endometrium. As implantation occurs the pre-embryo manufactures a hormone – human chorionic gonadotropin (HCG). It is this hormone that is the basis for pregnancy tests.

Once the sperm – about 200 million of them – have been deposited high in the vagina by the penis, their fate depends on the acidity of the vagina and the mucus of the cervix. The sperm are guided by the mucus into cervical reservoirs (*crypts*) where they will be stored, and released in batches to the uterus.

During this time the sperm are relatively inactive. They go through a process known as *capacitation* – acquiring the ability to stick to and penetrate the egg. If intercourse has occurred 48 hours prior to ovulation, the chance of fertilization taking place is good. From the uterus, the sperm that have survived the journey so far are moved by uterine contractions to the fallopian tubes. By this stage there may only be 200 sperm, and of those, only a few get through to the ampulla waiting to rendezvous with the egg which will remain in its fertile state for about 24 hours.

It is not known how or why just one sperm meets with and is able to penetrate the egg. Perhaps it is one of those wonderful mysteries of life that should always remain that way, for it is this meeting and merging that determines what sex your baby will be, his or her looks, health, personality, talents, and each one of his or her attributes.

The sperm has to penetrate the outer zone of the egg, and once this occurs the egg becomes impenetrable to other sperm – a swift, highly complex series of events. But fertilization doesn't end there – the full procedure takes about 24 hours, during which time the first cell division takes place and the egg begins the journey described above through the fallopian tubes and into the uterus.

So, there we have a simplistic look at an incredibly complex procedure, and when it works with the delicate, clock-like precision that nature intended, it will make a baby.

3

What Can Go Wrong Physically?

There are many different causes of fertility problems, and sometimes more than one factor can affect the man or the woman. It may be that both partners have a very minor problem. For example, the man may have a marginally low sperm count, and his partner may be in her late thirties and past her reproductive prime. The combination of these two factors could be enough to cause a fertility problem.

By the time a couple approach a natural therapist, they have usually already had all the preliminary tests done. Often no cause can be found for the problem. This diagnosis is not terribly satisfactory – every couple wants to know why they cannot conceive. Couples often come to natural therapy with a sense of frustration and hopelessness.

The perspective of the natural health practitioner, however, is quite different. From an acupuncture, naturopathic and osteopathic point of view such a diagnosis simply shows an imbalance of the body's biochemistry, energy flows or structural problems and once the underlying conditions are corrected, the fertility problem is usually resolved. What is more, you feel completely revitalized, and symptoms unrelated to fertility also disappear because you are enjoying better general health.

This chapter looks at the physical factors that affect fertility and considers some of the reasons why a pregnancy cannot be achieved or maintained.

The Causes of Subfertility in a Woman

The following are all factors that can affect the ability of a woman to reproduce:

- hormonal imbalances;
- ovarian disease;
- endometriosis;
- pelvic inflammatory disease (PID);
- cervical problems;

- uterine fibroids, adhesions and polyps;
- ectopic pregnancy;
- miscarriage;
- age;
- weight.

Hormonal Imbalances

We noted in Chapter 2 that hormones control the workings of our reproductive system. Not surprisingly, hormonal imbalances are frequently the cause of conditions that lead to female subfertility. Imbalances can be the result of endocrine diseases such as diabetes. Or the problem may lie with the adrenal glands, the thyroid glands, the ovaries, the corpus luteum, or the hypothalamic–pituitary system.

Other causes of hormone imbalances are the Pill, nutritional deficiencies, eating disorders, excessive exercise, stress, depression, medication and toxic exposure.

Hormonal imbalances can manifest themselves in problems such as an irregular menstrual cycle, the absence of menstrual periods and cessation of ovulation, the lack of cervical mucus, or a defective corpus luteum causing an inadequate luteal phase of the cycle. If the luteal phase is insufficient, infertility or miscarriage results. Severe pain before or during your period (dysmenorrhoea) and profuse bleeding (menorrhagia), can also be symptoms of a hormone imbalance. The causes of either of these symptoms must be checked.

Nutrition, mineral therapy, herbs and acupuncture are particularly good in helping to balance endocrine function, and therefore restoring hormone balance.

Ovulation factors account for 25 per cent of fertility problems. A normal period is the result of ovulation. Irregular periods, medically known as oligomenorrhoea, indicate infrequent ovulation or lack of ovulation (anovulation). Normal menstrual periods have a cycle of 28–29 days and menstruation is produced by decreasing progesterone levels, with little variation in the length and heaviness of the menstrual flow from one cycle to the next. Anovulatory menstrual periods are triggered by fluctuating oestrogen levels. They vary in length and heaviness from one cycle to another, are usually painless and occur after intervals of six weeks or more.

The absence of menstrual periods, known as amenorrhoea, is

diagnosed after six months without periods, and indicates that ovulation is not taking place. If you have missed your periods for several months, you should have a pregnancy test to ensure you are not pregnant; an early menopause should also be tested for. If neither test is positive, then the cause of the amenorrhoea must be determined and corrected.

If Hormone Replacement Therapy (HRT) is used to correct a hormone imbalance, often the underlying cause remains uncorrected and further imbalances can result.

Ovarian Disease

Polycystic Ovary Disease (PCOD) accounts for approximately 6 per cent of ovulation problems. It occurs when too much luteinizing hormone (LH) and testosterone is produced, and too little follicle stimulating hormone (FSH). The ovaries develop multiple cysts (follicles) and can become enlarged, inhibiting normal follicle development and ovulation. Symptoms include weight gain and infrequent periods and sometimes also acne and excess body and facial hair.

PCOD is very difficult to treat, but most cases respond to natural therapies. However, it will take many months to correct. Your treatment should incorporate mineral therapy, acupuncture, and herbs, some of which must be avoided in pregnancy. If herbs are part of your treatment you must use a condom while treating PCOD.

Ovarian cysts are not to be confused with PCOD. They are usually small and benign, causing little or no trouble and usually disappear spontaneously. Generally symptoms are pain during ovulation, menstruation or intercourse. However sometimes they can rupture, in which case pain is severe. Occasionally cysts grow rapidly, or turn malignant. If you have cause for concern check with your healthcare professional. Small uncomplicated cysts generally respond well to mineral therapy and herbs.

Endometriosis

Endometriosis is an extremely painful and often debilitating condition where tissue and blood identical to the uterine lining grow outside the uterus. This 'rogue' tissue, which responds to hormonal changes just as the uterine lining does, breaks down and bleeds during the menstrual period. As the blood cannot escape it bleeds into the surrounding tissues and organs. Scarring (adhesions) can result, and if scars develop on the outside of the tubes near the ovary, the 'fingers' on the tube ends may have difficulty picking up the egg to set it on its journey through the tube.

High oestrogen levels are a cause of endometriosis. Impaired lymphatic function can result in pelvic congestion and the liver function may not be sufficient to conjugate and eliminate oestrogen. A lowered immune system may not recognize and destroy misplaced endometrial cells. It is suspected that environmental toxins may also be a factor, as is stress, which results in exhaustion and general debility.

Besides infertility, symptoms of endometriosis can include severe period pain, painful intercourse, pelvic pain, pain on urinating or defecating, intestinal discomfort, and menstrual irregularity.

Endometriosis responds well to natural treatments. Mineral therapy and dietary changes are usually successful used alone. If herbal remedies, homoeopathy or acupuncture are used, these should be as an adjunct to mineral therapy.

Pelvic Inflammatory Disease

Pelvic Inflammatory Disease (PID) accounts for 35 per cent of fertility problems. It is an infection of the uterus, cervix and ovaries. When the tubes are affected, the condition is known as *salpingitis*, which can result in blocked or damaged tubes. Microsurgery can in some cases reverse tube blockage.

Complications from an IUD or pelvic surgery can result in PID. However, the main cause is sexually transmitted diseases such as gonorrhoea, chlamydia, mycoplasmas, or, rarely, systemic candida. If sexually transmitted diseases are not treated, infertility, not subfertility, will result. There is a 50 per cent chance of recurrence, 33 per cent chance of sterility, 25 per cent chance of pain on intercourse, and a 10 per cent chance of ectopic pregnancy if no treatment is sought.

In some cases of PID there are no noticeable symptoms until the disease is well advanced and may already have caused fertility problems, such as inflammation and consequent adhesions or tube damage. These can disrupt the organic function of the tube destroying the fine muscle structure and the tiny cilia that help propel the egg along the microscopically narrow passage. It can also increase your chances of an ectopic pregnancy. Symptoms of PID may include fever, severe lower abdominal pain and pelvic swelling, and abnormal vaginal discharge or irregular vaginal bleeding may occur. If you have any cause to suspect you may have PID you should contact your doctor immediately.

Orthodox treatment, that is antibiotics specific to the infection, must be used together with acupuncture, herbal remedies or homoeopathy, and should resolve this condition if treated early enough. If the immune system is strengthened there may be less chance of relapse. A sound nutritional programme must therefore be part of any successful treatment.

Cervical Problems

A healthy cervix, in response to hormones, produces mucus that changes throughout the cycle, denoting infertile and fertile days (see Chapter 5). A poorly functioning cervix will produce inadequate cervical mucus that will not be able to nurture and help transport the sperm through the uterus to the fallopian tubes.

Problems may result from surgery such as a cone biopsy or other treatments to the cervix. You should follow up any cervical treatment with mineral therapy, antioxidants and herbs.

The mucus itself may be too acidic. If so, the condition is easily and quickly treated with mineral therapy and diet. You can purchase pH sticks from your pharmacy to check the reduction in the acidity of the mucus during treatment.

You may have antibodies that immobilize the sperm. Again, this condition generally responds well to treatment. If either you or your partner has an antibody problem, use condoms for three months. During this time a full nutritional programme including allergy avoidance must be followed. After this time, your first unprotected intercourse should take place just prior to ovulation.

Cervical incompetence, where the cervix is unable to support a foetus, is generally not noticed until a pregnancy terminates at about 14 weeks. Symptoms that may indicate you have this problem are backache and a vaginal wetness or discharge. You should contact your specialist immediately if you notice any of these symptoms. A cervical stitch could save your baby.

Mineral therapy is a good supporting treatment here, but it is important to begin a full nutritional programme four months prior to trying for a conception.

Uterine Fibroids, Adhesions and Polyps

Fibroids, adhesions and polyps may cause problems, depending on how their growth affects the uterus. Fibroids, which are benign growths of the uterine wall, occur in approximately one third of women over the age of 35. They are caused by high oestrogen levels and can be just a few millimetres in size, or fill the entire abdominal cavity. Symptoms that may indicate the presence of fibroids are painful periods, excessive bleeding, a whitish, yellowish discharge from the vagina, and sometimes backache.

Fibroids are difficult to treat. Most women don't know they have them until they are big enough to cause a problem. A natural therapy approach is going to take time and may not always be successful. Fibroids can be surgically removed, and in some instances a hysterectomy may need to be carried out.

Adhesions can cause amenorrhoea and prevent a pregnancy occurring. Treatment depends on how badly damaged the endometrium is. If small and 'young' they can often be 'melted' with natural treatments. If severe, surgery will be necessary. Acupuncture and osteopathy are also good for this problem.

Polyps are benign growths, and are best dealt with surgically. However, as they are inclined to recur, a nutritional programme including the minerals used to treat fibroids should help.

If your uterus is retroverted, don't worry. It will not prevent you conceiving and carrying your baby.

Ectopic Pregnancy

An ectopic pregnancy can occur as a result of abnormalities of the fallopian tubes, the uterus, or any condition which interferes with normal implantation such as adhesions or polyps. Other causes of ectopic pregnancies are assisted conception, previous infertility, or PID. The pregnancy usually occurs in the fallopian tube, but other sites are the abdomen, and, rarely, the ovaries or cervix.

Symptoms of an ectopic pregnancy are discomfort and pain which can be severe and may or may not be localized to the right or left of the lower abdomen or pelvis. There may be internal bleeding, haemorrhage and symptoms of shock. Extreme weakness and fainting can occur. There may be pain in one or both shoulders and a bluish tinge of the umbilicus. A pregnancy test may not show a positive reading, so if you suspect something is wrong, do not hesitate to contact your specialist, as surgery must be carried out immediately.

Miscarriage

Miscarriage is sometimes known as spontaneous abortion and occurs in approximately 12 per cent of pregnancies in women younger than 20, increasing to 13 per cent in the 20–24 age group, and to 16 per cent in the 30–34 age group. There is a 25 per cent chance of miscarrying if you are between 40 and 42, and a 50 per cent chance if you are 43 or older. The eggs diminish in quality as a woman gets older, and the likelihood of miscarriage increases.

It is estimated that one third of all pregnancies end without the mother knowing she is pregnant, but thinking she is having a heavier than usual or slightly delayed period. The cause is most likely to be an imperfect embryo. Once a pregnancy has been established, most miscarriages occur within the first 12 weeks of pregnancy. The problem may be with the embryo itself; other factors include ovulation, a hormonal imbalance affecting the endometrium, problems with the uterus or cervix, diseases of the fallopian tubes, or endometriosis.

Medical treatment will depend on the kind of miscarriage suffered and when it occurs in the pregnancy. But for the couple concerned there is only one kind of miscarriage – tragic. A dilatation and curettage (D & C) is usually performed where the cervix is dilated and the lining of the uterus scraped with a curette to ensure no tissue is left behind that could be a source of infection.

If you have had the misfortune to experience a miscarriage you must ensure that you are well and truly over it, and have spent four to six months getting yourself to optimum health before attempting another pregnancy. Miscarriages are not just bad luck or 'chance' occurrences. They can often be prevented with good nutrition that helps balance the hormones and produce healthy sperm and eggs. If miscarriage does threaten, then rest and phone your specialist and natural health practitioner. Ideally these two caregivers should work together for optimum benefit to you.

Miscarriage is a terrible kind of suffering no matter how early on in the pregnancy it occurs, partly because the mother and father have lost a baby they have never known. Sometimes couples will not talk about their grief. Often the father senses the loss every bit as much as the mother, yet he feels he has to be 'strong' for his partner's sake. While everybody comforts the mother, the father is often completely overlooked. Talking must be encouraged. If you know a couple who have experienced a miscarriage, never fob off the tragedy with the comment, 'Don't worry, you can have another one.' That lost baby will remain in the parents' hearts and minds all their lives.

Robyn's story
I married at 21. At 27 I had a miscarriage. At 38 we began thinking we would never get to be a mum and dad. I began a simple natural treatment of minerals along with dietary changes. I was told to visualize my tubes and uterus opening to greet and hold our baby. A bit strange, but we both began this little mental exercise. During my next cycle I conceived. We now have a beautiful healthy baby.

Age

Age is the single most important cause of fertility problems in women. Couples today do not think of starting families until the woman is older. The demands and structure of today's society do not make it easy for couples to start their family while the woman is still in her twenties when her reproductive health is at its best. Couples want to feel financially secure before bringing a baby into the world, or to have completed their education or training, to have travelled, or established a career.

However, if you wait too long, then you can have trouble conceiving. A healthy man remains fertile for much of his life. A woman is at the height of her fertile years from the mid- to late twenties. From the age of 30, the quality of the eggs declines, and from 40 onwards the uterus loses its integrity, making it difficult to maintain a pregnancy.

Another factor that most people are aware of is that older women are more likely to suffer chromosomal defects, which may result in a baby with Down's syndrome, a condition also linked to nutritional deficiencies. There are medical tests available to show the body's chromosomal patterns – and your doctor may suggest this as a routine check.

A healthy, well-nourished body is the key to older women having a healthy pregnancy and a healthy baby.

Claire's story

In my twenties I had a wonderful job that took me to many different countries. I married at 30 and when my husband was granted a fellowship in the States, I decided to further my post-graduate education. Babies somehow didn't enter the picture.

When I was 41 I woke up one morning and suddenly realized we all have a biological clock. I wanted a baby. We both wanted a baby – suddenly, desperately.

A friend of mine was a naturopath. She advised me to come off the Pill immediately, but not to get pregnant for at least four months, preferably six. It seemed an eternity. I was put on a simple formula of minerals, essential fatty acids, and vitamins, including folic acid. At 42 I had a perfectly formed beautiful daughter after a perfect pregnancy.

I felt so good on the nutritional supplements I maintained a basic daily regime – I wanted to give the best I could to motherhood. At 44 I became pregnant again. After another good pregnancy, our son – perfect and beautiful – was born.

Maybe I would have been lucky without any help – but at my age I was not prepared to chance it. Our children are now ten and eight. They are healthy, happy, and we have never had behavioural or educational problems with them.

Anne's story

I married at 37, and four years later we still had not achieved a pregnancy. I was aware of the Foresight programme and knew a naturopath who worked in a similar way.

My treatment consisted of a personally assessed mineral formula, and vitamins. My diet, which was pretty good anyway, was checked for allergens. Within a month I began feeling subtly different and I had more energy. Three months later I was pregnant. It was a textbook pregnancy. Kirsten was just two when I became pregnant again, and Andre followed after another good pregnancy. The children are now 13 and 11. They are healthy, have good scholastic records and are fun to be with.

Weight

While women ideally should carry more fat than men, overweight women (and men) are less fertile. In the case of women, if you are too thin, you may not produce sufficient oestrogen, or if you carry too much fat, your progesterone production may be inhibited. A change in your weight may result in cycle irregularities. You can achieve your ideal weight with dietary reform and a sensible exercise programme. If you have had an eating disorder in the past, you will be deficient in some key nutrients, and this should always be addressed. If you are overweight, even a small weight loss is very likely to improve ovulation, which in turn will enhance the chances of falling pregnant.

Causes of Subfertility in a Man

Many men do not consider they are important enough to be part of a treatment programme. Usually, by the time couples come to a natural practitioner, a sperm count has already been carried out. If it is all right, the man often feels he need do nothing more. However, an assessment of nutritional deficiencies and masked allergies is vital. Other specific tests may also need to be done. Even if the prospective father considers himself to be in excellent health, this must be assessed at cell level. The father is, after all, half of the baby-making equation.

The support a man gives to his partner during the initial consultation with a natural therapy practitioner is something only he can offer. It is traumatic for the prospective mother to go through her case history yet again to another 'new' person. It is now common for practitioners working in the fertility field to request both partners attend the initial consultation. If a couple wants the best chance for conception, a healthy pregnancy and a baby, both partners must take part in the programme. Nothing should be left to chance when you are considering bringing a baby into the world. It is a huge responsibility that rests with both parents.

The following are physical factors that affect the fertility of a man:

- low sperm count, poor motility, and 'clumping';
- anti-sperm antibodies;
- defects in the coital technique;
- erectile dysfunction;
- elevated scrotal temperature.

Low Sperm Count, Poor Motility, and 'Clumping'

Low sperm counts are the major cause of male subfertility, yet medically no cause can be found for 90 per cent of cases. The sperm are extremely fragile and vulnerable to many different factors, including environmental pollutants, diet and lifestyle. Over the past 50 years sperm counts in a normal ejaculation have fallen by almost half. The quality of the sperm is also diminishing – sperm motility is declining and the proportion of abnormal sperm in the ejaculate is increasing. Sperm health is more important than quantity, although there is a correlation between sperm numbers and fertility.

Exposure to Diethylsteilbesterol (DES) or other forms of oestrogen during gestation can cause a low sperm count, diminished semen volume and other disorders of the male urino-genital system.

Sperm counts can be temporarily reduced by exposure to radiation, organochlorines and heavy metals, and also by some prescription drugs; by alcohol, tobacco and other social drugs; and by illness, stress and fatigue. Men who have jobs that require long periods of sitting or driving tend to have low sperm counts.

Acupuncture, osteopathy and boosting nutrient levels to correct the biochemistry of the body can help increase sperm count and enhance sperm health.

Tony's story

For nine years we suffered alone. While all our friends were having children nothing was happening for us. For two years I had been working with a urologist trying to raise my sperm count. Nothing happened. Tess, my wife, mentioned our problem to a naturopath she went to and she was told, well for a start, no tight underpants, get off the hormones, and get him to take a magnesium formula and zinc. I did this for two months, then I thought, if we are going to do this, let's do it properly, so I had more minerals and a few vitamins (this time prescribed), and in five months we achieved a pregnancy. One daughter was followed by another soon after. They are now beautiful young women.

Marc's story

I come from a background where the man is never at fault if a couple can't produce a baby. My partner was found to be normal and I was asked to have a sperm count done. I was shattered to find that not only was my sperm count low, but I had a lot of abnormal sperm and would probably never father a child. I didn't know who to turn to. I started to read up on the subject and found sperm health could be improved with nutrition.

I talked to a naturopath. She pointed out that my previous jobs had involved working with pesticides and commercial cleaning compounds. These I had worked with for six years. She advised no smoking or alcohol. I was put on a mixture of potassium, magnesium, silica, sodium sulphate, zinc and manganese, selenium, an essential fatty acid, vitamin B complex and vitamins A, C and E. All these were worked out according to my individual needs and would help elevate my sperm count and help my body detoxify residual chemical molecules.

I learned that as the sperm took 100 days to develop and mature, I should not expect too much too soon. Acupuncture was also discussed and would be used if necessary. My partner also took supplements and we had various tests. That was a long year. There were times when I thought I would give up, but as I went on with the treatment my overall health improved and I realized I had not felt so well for many years. Nine months later my wife conceived and we now have a daughter.

Anti-sperm Antibodies

Anti-sperm antibodies are usually the sign of a past or present infection. The antibodies can cause sperm to 'clump' or impede their movement and ability to penetrate the cervical mucus. Chlamydia is the most common sexually transmitted disease (STD), causing inflammation of the prostate, rectum, testes and scarring or blockage of the epididymis and vas deferens. Sterility or impaired sperm production can result. Men can remain symptom-free after contact for years. Or pain may be experienced in the pelvic area or scrotum, and with urinating or ejaculation. There may also be a penal discharge.

If you suspect you are infected with chlamydia, gonorrhoea or any other infection, have it checked immediately. The consequences for the male and the female of STDs are horrendous.

STDs must be treated with antibiotics, ideally in conjunction with natural treatments that help boost immunity and prevent any recurrence.

Defects in the Coital Technique

Coital problems are something that no man feels he should have, or own up to. If premature withdrawal, premature ejaculation or your coital technique is the cause or part of the cause of the fertility problem, the quicker you discuss it with a specialist sex therapist, the quicker conception can become a reality. But never let intercourse become a technicality, and never lose sight of the fact that it is the ultimate expression of love. There is no best position for conception. Whatever is most enjoyable and comfortable for you is fine, provided the ejaculate is deposited high up in the vagina, close to the cervix. It is not abnormal if some of the semen leaks from the vagina. It has been observed that female orgasm occurring prior to ejaculation decreases sperm retention, and orgasm after ejaculation increases sperm retention.

Erectile Dysfunction

Erectile dysfunction or impotence can be caused by alcohol, tobacco, vascular insufficiency, hormonal imbalances, diabetes, hypothyroidism, multiple sclerosis, prostate or penal disorders and pelvic surgery. Stress, depression and anxiety can also be causes, and if you worry about achieving or maintaining an erection, it may only make the condition worse. Sometimes impotence has a deep psychological cause.

Some medication can also cause erectile dysfunction and low sperm counts. Prescription medicines such as antihistamines, antidepressants, tranquillizers, and antihypertensives all influence the availability of specific nutrients, and while you should never think of abandoning any medical treatment suddenly and without professional advice, most of the conditions that these drugs are taken for can be corrected naturally.

> *Approximately 30 per cent of male fertility problems are caused by coital technique or by erectile dysfunction.*

Nutrition is important, and herbs and acupuncture can also help. If the problem is psychological, consulting a counsellor is a good way to help you overcome the difficulty. The sooner you pursue this the quicker you will overcome the problem.

Elevated Scrotal Temperature

Elevated scrotal temperature can also inhibit the production of sperm. Sperm are housed within the scrotum, but even the scrotum can get too hot, especially if you wear tight clothing such as jeans, underwear or synthetic sportswear. Hot baths can also cause a rise in scrotal temperature.

If you wear tight underwear, go trendy and become a boxershort buff. If you have to wear synthetic sportswear, do not stay in the gear any longer than necessary, and ensure you wear cotton (or silk) at other times. After exercise, let the scrotum hang free to allow the temperature to return to normal. If you like to have hot baths or saunas, don't stay in for more than six minutes; and afterwards give the scrotal area a cool blast with the shower or have a cool sitz bath.

Varicoceles are varicose veins that can be seen through the fine skin of the scrotum. These can also elevate your temperature. If they are not too bad, then natural therapies may be able to improve or stabilize the problem. If they are severe, then you will need to have them surgically removed.

4

Other Factors Affecting Fertility

This chapter looks at causes of fertility problems that are not directly related to physical factors. It deals with the psychological reasons for difficulties in conceiving, and also looks at food and diet, allergies, hormonal supplements and environmental factors.

Fertility and the Mind

When it comes to identifying causes of fertility problems, medical experts seldom consider the link between the body and the mind. Although several medical studies have shown that couples who adopt a child do not have increased chances of conceiving, many readers will know of women who have tried to conceive for several years (and have often given up), and who have then had a child after adopting a baby or starting to work with children. It may be that working with children changes the link between the body and the mind sufficiently to stimulate the reproductive hormones. Or perhaps being more relaxed provides the necessary trigger – couples may feel they need not 'try' so hard after they have adopted a baby. Psychological factors are not easy to pinpoint.

Some research has been done on the links between depression and fertility. One study found that the hormones released under stress can adversely affect the reproductive system. We commonly hear stories of how a trauma or great sadness has caused an early menopause, or periods becoming irregular or stopping for some months. But even a mild depression or negative feelings can affect fertility.

Michelle's story

My natural therapy practitioner told me I must change my mind-set. I was so negative. We went over the things that were causing me to be so sad – apart from the baby issue. I just kept thinking I will never be pregnant. I hated my job, so I changed it. I hated the way our friends kept asking when we were going to have children, so we avoided them and mixed only with those whom we felt really understood our problem, and never asked questions. With treatment we both feel we are doing all we can. I feel more positive about the future, whether or not we have children.

Negative feelings can be hard to avoid

I feel I am not a complete woman, not being able to have a child.
Joan

I feel so inadequate.
Andy

Being called an empty vessel is one thing. To feel that emptiness is another. We are considering fostering, as we are both in our forties now. At least that way we could give something to the community.
Gavin

Not being able to have the baby you desperately want can be stressful in itself. Staying relaxed makes it easier to conceive, yet not becoming pregnant can trigger stress and lock you into a vicious psychological circle. Couples undergoing assisted conception are particularly prone to stress. They find the procedure wrecks sex, as they start to see themselves as baby-making machines. It is important to keep on loving each other at times like this and to keep the romance in the relationship.

Sometimes couples experience problems when one partner's interest in sex varies greatly from the other's. It may be helpful in this context to think of levels of sexual activity on a continuum. At one end of the continuum are the *hyper-sexual*, those for whom the sexual urge is so strong it becomes compulsive and interferes with day-to-day life. At the other end are the *hypo-sexual*, those who have no interest in or an aversion to sexual activity, who have no dreams or fantasies. The majority of people fall somewhere in the middle of the continuum. But if you are at either extreme, it could be a sign of severe stress that is not being dealt with. If one partner is significantly higher or lower than the other on the continuum, then the couple are likely to suffer psychological problems and will need to explore ways of overcoming their difficulties, perhaps with the help of a counsellor or sex therapist.

There may be some conflict or lack of clarity about whether or not to have children.

John wants a child. I don't. I wonder if we should continue our relationship.
Kerry

I don't think I really want a baby, but we are continually being asked when we are going to start a family. It gets to you in the end. You feel you have to have a child.
Jo

The causes of psychological difficulties can be deeply ingrained. Childhood experiences can affect us in powerful ways in our adult years, and often they are related to feelings of fear. Some couples have a fear of being a parent, or are afraid of what a baby might do to the relationship or lifestyle. Some women are afraid of pregnancy or birth.

My mother died following my birth. I suppose I was so frightened of giving birth myself it never happened.
Nola, now aged 60

There may be other experiences from childhood or early adult years that have remained unresolved in our minds – our 'unfinished business'. For instance, issues of abuse or guilt may not have been properly dealt with.

I had an abortion when I was 21. I am sure I will never have another child.
Nina

I gave up a daughter for adoption when I was 16. After 13 years of trying for a pregnancy, my partner and I still had no children. We had had five goes at IVF. Then I heard from my daughter who wanted to meet me. One year after she came into my life, I had the first of our two children.
Jenni

At times the 'unfinished business' can relate to unfulfilled hopes and aspirations. The woman may wish to secure a career before embarking on motherhood, or one partner may have ambitions that conflict with parenting.

Diane and Grant's story
Diane (28) and Grant (30) wanted to become parents. She was depressed that after seven years of trying to conceive nothing had happened. On her third monthly visit she came without Grant and confided that she would like to go overseas for one year. So intense

28

was this desire she said she would sell the house to finance it. Grant knew nothing about her wish to travel. I suggested this might be why a pregnancy had not occurred. Diane eventually did go overseas, without selling their home, and six years later I met them with two beautiful little girls who had been conceived without any help at all.

If you feel your problem could be psychological, you must talk with your partner in total honesty. Ask if you want a baby for the right reasons, not just because it seems to be the right thing to do, according to your friends or family. Do you *both* want a baby? Is there something within your relationship that is troubling you? Or something you fear? It is important to talk about it. Look at yourselves honestly and seek help from a specialist psychotherapist. Therapy can be very rewarding.

What You Eat

There are many reasons why our sources of food are proving deficient in terms of nutrition. Farming practices have scant regard for nurturing the soil and working with nature. As a result, the nutrient value of meat, vegetables, fruits and grains has become grossly altered and depleted. The trend towards eating processed food has increased greatly over the past 50 years. We ingest a huge number of chemicals which can cause deficiencies and affect our hormones.

Our ancestors existed on a natural diet of unprocessed complex carbohydrates and lightly cooked protein. One third of their intake consisted of protein in the form of meat from animals that roamed over and ate grasses that had not been top dressed; in coastal areas, fish and seaweeds were eaten. The remaining two thirds of the diet comprised raw and lightly cooked green leafy vegetables and herbs, lightly cooked vegetables including roots and tubers, and in smaller amounts grains, pulses, fruits, nuts and seeds. Spices, honey, naturally fermented vinegar and alcohol, the latter two high in enzymes, were used in moderation as seasonings. Where milk products were used the milk was usually soured (clabbered) to give a yoghurt-like product that was more easily tolerated than current-day pasteurized and homogenized products.

It seems that the further we transgress from a whole, natural food diet, containing lots of raw vegetables and fruit and lightly cooked protein, the more our health and fertility will suffer. The following table, based on the research of Burkitt and Trowell in the 1970s, shows how changes in diet have affected human health since the industrial revolution, but particularly since the early 1900s, which marked the beginnings of the commercialization of food production. If Burkitt and Trowell were working today, they would add Stage Five – fertility problems and babies born with compromised health.

FOUR STAGES OF THE CHANGES IN DIET AND HEALTH

Stage	Type of Diet	State of Health
One	Natural diet consisting mainly of unprocessed complex carbohydrates (plants)	Few of the diseases and health problems now common in modern society
Two	Introduction of commercial Western diet – refined carbohydrates, saturated fats and processed foods	Obesity, diabetes observed among the more affluent
Three	Increase of processed refined and 'fast' foods	Common occurrence of constipation, haemorrhoids, varicose veins, appendicitis
Four	Full 'Westernization' of diet	Prevalence of ischemic heart disease, diverticular disease, hiatal hernia, cancer

FROM BURKITT AND TROWELL

The trace mineral content of the hunter/gatherer diet was markedly higher than and in different proportions to the modern Western diet. Sodium intake was less than one quarter. Calcium was at least double that of our modern diet. Bones were included in stew-type dishes or soups, and some peoples added a dash of vinegar to release the calcium into the stock. Ninety per cent of magnesium, along with vitamins B and E, is now lost through modern milling processes.

The fibre or roughage content of their food was nearly ten times that of our modern, highly refined diet. Fruits, vegetables, whole-grains, nuts, seeds, seaweeds and pulses were eaten in their natural state, giving a complex of polysaccharides, cellulose, hemicelluloses, gums, mucilages, lignins along with associated nutrients. Very few of these nutrients are present in the refined flour and sugar that make up a huge portion of our modern-day daily food intake.

The meat we eat today has approximately 50 per cent more fat which yields a high content of unhealthy saturated fatty acids and none of the important essential fatty acids that the earlier leaner animals did.

The hunter/gatherer diet is the kind that naturopaths still try to work with today, in a modern context, of course. While I am not advocating we return to pulling raw food apart with our fingers, I do recommend trying to reintroduce the principles of a real wholefood diet into our daily eating programmes.

Food Additives

Paying attention to the food we eat and how we grow it only partly addresses the problem of diet. With modern manufacturing practices, nearly four thousand additives have been introduced to our food chain. Some of these are mutagens that not only damage and kill living cells, but react with our chromosomes and genes that carry our genetic code. Damage from mutagens is greatest in the weeks prior to conception and in early pregnancy.

It is estimated that each person consumes 3.5–4.5 kg of additives per year. We are told these chemicals are safe, but I do not know of any study that accurately indicates the danger or safety of the metabolites of the chemicals once they are ingested, or the results of a 'cocktail' of these chemicals.

Natural Foods

As soon as a food is tampered with in any way it is no longer 'natural'. Once food manufacturing started to become big business, we seemed to lose our reverence for food as 'the source of life'. The 'natural' produce we buy through the supermarkets or fruit and vegetable outlets is usually commercially grown in soil that is deficient in minerals because it has been overworked and treated with artificial fertilizers. The produce is sprayed with pesticides, fungicides, and herbicides, all of which become part of the soil and the tissue of the produce grown.

> About 90 per cent of the organochlorine toxicity our bodies are subjected to daily comes from the food we eat.

It is not only during cultivation that foods are subject to a barrage of toxins. Once foods are harvested, processed or packaged they and their containers can be sprayed with a variety of 'protective' chemicals to prevent sprouting and storage-related diseases or damage. Gases are used to control ripening. Grains are sprayed with pesticides, with the result that anything made with flour, or flour itself, contains toxins. Wholegrains and wheat bran in particular have a high residual pesticide count.

Our animals today are usually farmed with chemicals, hormones, and antibiotics. Some of these are mixed with their food which can consist of factors unnatural to their digestive system. Once corn comes on-line as cattle feed, it is usual for scraps such as paper and cardboard, complete with chemicals from the inks and glues or plastic used in their manufacture, and other cellulose-containing scrap products to be added to the food mix. The animals will consequently yield meat that contains metabolites of antibiotics, hormones and toxins from such food.

Hormones are used to speed growth in animals. Many health professionals have encountered patients with hormone problems, which after medical investigations were 'attributed probably to beef treated with hormones'. Animals that have been fed hormones can affect our health in a variety of ways. For example, certain sheep dips have become not only part of the meat we eat, but the wool our carpets and clothes are made from. If a chicken is 'free-range' it is worth knowing whether it has been given dried food with added antibiotics and hormones. Although we are only exposed to small traces of these chemicals, in combination they become a potentially dangerous cocktail overloading our systems and affecting our hormones.

Genetically Modified Foods

Although genetically modified seed produces crops that appear almost identical to the unmodified product, we simply cannot predict the long-term effect on human health. There are also concerns about the long-term effect on the environment. 'Food safe' does not mean 'ecology safe'. In one experiment where potatoes were modified to become toxic to aphids, the ladybirds eating those aphids as part of their natural foods died. Researchers cannot explain why. What are the implications for the food chain as a whole? Once genetically modified crops are in the environment, they cannot be withdrawn.

Six chemical companies dominate the international seed market. Genetically altered seeds are in existence for crops that provide the world with 90 per cent of its foods. These are potato, soy, corn, sugarbeet and cotton, plus wheat, rice and other crops, which are currently under experimentation. Already it is possible to buy an increasing number of foods containing genetically altered ingredients such as soy from genetically altered beans. Some of these are being sold as 'health' foods. As the law currently stands, manufacturers are not required to label foods containing genetically modified products. However, many foods are now appearing with the simple words 'GM free'.

Irradiation

Irradiation is a superb sterilization procedure for medical equipment. That is what it was devised for, and where it should stay. Unfortunately, the stage is set for irradiated foods to be sold. Foods targeted are likely to be meats, herbs, spices, fruit, vegetables, especially potatoes, onions and grains.

When foods or products undergo irradiation, the electrons in the food's naturally occurring chemicals are knocked out of orbit; molecular rearrangement occurs, and free radicals are formed. Irradiated foods which are 'off' have no warning smell. Aflotoxin, a mould-producing carcinogen, is produced in higher quantities. Disease-producing organisms can mutate, and more chemicals have to be used to counteract changes in texture, smell, and flavour as a result of this process. Most vitamins and some amino acids are depleted or destroyed. Carbohydrates create new toxic chemicals, none of which has been adequately tested.

The Allergy Factor

Allergies compromise your general health, and compromised health compromises fertility. An allergy is a reflection of the way we eat. Allergies occur when the antigen (offending food) provokes an antibody reaction which releases chemicals such as histamine in our bodies. These 'mediators' or chemical imbalances cause a dysfunction of our immune system and the occurrence of abnormal cellular reactions. Various systems of the body can be affected, including the nervous system and muscles. Allergies can produce an inflammation, an over-production of mucus, or cause digestive disturbances that affect nutrient uptake. The blood flow can slow, causing symptoms such as brain fag or 'spaciness', headaches or migraines. Hormones can also be affected. Some of the allergy symptoms and reactions described above have a direct influence on fertility.

Allergies can be caused by many different factors:

- eating one food or group of foods too much too often;
- early weaning, and foods being given too young in life;
- altered foods provoking reactions between food molecules and normal tissue; most foods have been 'altered' in some way, and apart from organic food, all have been contaminated with toxins;
- food eaten in concentrated form, such as orange in the form of juice, or tomatoes as a puree;
- familial predisposition. Some families are more inclined towards allergies than others, but the foods causing the allergy (allergens) may vary;
- being frequently exposed to or exposed at an early age to allergenic substances, or dust and pollens.

Allergies may be 'fixed', if you have an immediate response to a food or environmental allergen, or 'masked'. A fixed allergy can be dangerous if you have a sudden violent reaction; however, the masked or hidden allergy is what causes chronic health problems and may adversely affect reproduction. It will certainly compromise the health of your future baby. Chronic symptoms that require ongoing medication are very often the result of an allergy. Eliminate the allergy and you often overcome the need for daily medication, which can in turn deplete your nutrient balance and affect fertility.

Common masked allergens are dairy products, potatoes, tomatoes, soy, peanuts, citrus, eggs, chicken, wheat and sugar, coffee, tea, food additives and colouring.

Once the foods to which you are allergic are eliminated, your diet reformed, and your biochemistry balanced, you will find you will not react so distressingly to environmental 'triggers', such as dust, pollen and grasses, if these are a problem. Natural remedies will help you overcome distressing symptoms such as hayfever while your health is being improved.

If you know which foods you are allergic to, you must avoid that food totally while trying to conceive, while pregnant and during lactation. A four-day rotation of safe foods, and especially of the more common allergens, will give you a better chance of enhanced fertility, and do much to prevent your future baby being born allergic or developing allergies early in life.

Allergy management should be part of all good fertility treatment. Many natural health practitioners are skilled at allergy management. If not, they will refer you on.

Occasionally the symptoms of an allergy can be confused with those of candidiasis, an overgrowth of candida leading to an increased production of toxins. In this case, as soon as your allergens are avoided, your symptoms disappear. Candidiasis can also cause food allergies, as can nutrient deficiencies. Candidiasis is an over-diagnosed condition, but if you do suffer from it, then your practitioner will formulate your supplement regime and diet to balance your intestinal flora, which is part of a healthy gastro-intestinal tract. Symptoms of candidiasis can include fatigue, poor concentration, altered bowel habits, abdominal bloating, irritable bowel, itching of the anal or vulva area, and cravings. Because of its effect on mucus, candidiasis may make your cervical mucus hostile to sperm.

The Pill

It seems ironic to discuss the Pill in the context of fertility; however, many subfertility cases have been caused by this choice of contraception. The Pill works as a contraceptive by making the woman's mucus thick and sticky so the sperm cannot penetrate. The lining of the uterus grows wasted and thin, so it cannot support a pregnancy. It also stops you ovulating and stops normal menstruation. When you stop taking the Pill for a few days each month the bleed is a withdrawal bleed, not a real period.

The Pill can prevent the body returning to its normal hormonal pattern, and it can be months, sometimes years, before a menstrual cycle is resumed. In some cases it never returns. Natural treatments can correct this condition. Medically more hormones will be prescribed, but this treatment will not necessarily correct the underlying problems.

The Pill has many side effects, but those directly affecting fertility include:

- lowered resistance to infections including genito-urinary and fungal infections;
- ectopic pregnancy;
- mineral and vitamin imbalances;
- miscarriage, which can occur long after stopping the Pill unless the nutrient and hormonal levels have been corrected;
- cancer of the breast, uterus, liver and pituitary gland;
- food allergies.

The Pill is also associated with side effects that are important factors in pregnancy, including:

- hypertension;
- kidney failure;
- varicose veins;
- jaundice;
- blood sugar level disturbances;
- oedema;
- depression;
- weight gain;
- inhibited liver function;
- congenital malformations in offspring.

Nutritionally, the Pill raises copper and serum vitamin A levels and lowers magnesium, iron, iodine, zinc, vitamins B_1, B_2, B_3, B_6, B_{12}, folic acid and vitamin C. Chromium levels may also be affected.

Excess copper can be toxic and is associated with pre-eclampsia and post-natal depression.

Sylvia's story

When our second child was three, we decided to have another baby. I had been on the Pill for two years and six months following lactation. When I stopped taking it my periods didn't return, and nine months later my doctor suggested hormonal treatment. I thought hormones had made a big enough mess of my body, why should I take more? There had to be a different way, so I went natural. My periods returned three weeks into the treatment. We were told not to try to conceive for four months to give my body time to return to normal with nutritional treatment. I conceived five cycles after beginning treatment. We now use natural family planning.

Environmental Toxins

The developing sperm, egg, and foetus may be affected by exposure to environmental factors without you noticing any symptoms or having any obvious reactions. Exposure to environmental toxins, such as heavy metals, drugs, social poisons, radiation, and electro-magnetic fields have all been linked to fertility problems.

There are two main categories of environmental toxins:

- *Organophosphates* (OPs), which are water-soluble and generally break down quickly. They are acutely toxic to all mammals and primarily affect the central and autonomic nervous systems and the peripheral muscular pathways.
- *Organochlorines* (OCs), also known as xeno-oestrogens, chlorinated hydrocarbons or persistent organic pollutants (POPs), are not biodegradable. They remain in the soil and water supplies, never dispersing, and over time build up in the fatty tissue and liver of wildlife and humans.

Other chemicals or groups of chemicals commonly used in everyday products around the home, workplace and garden are carbamates, halogenated hydrocarbons, chlorinated phenoxy substances, hetero-cyclic compounds, phenolic compounds, amines, ureas, benzonitriles and pyrethroids (which should not be confused with the natural insecticide pyrethrum). Below is a list of items to check around the home and workplace for organochlorines. There are safe alternatives to most of these.

ITEMS IN THE HOME AND WORKPLACE THAT MIGHT CONTAIN ORGANOCHLORINES		
aerosols	fungicides	pipes
airconditioning	furniture	plastics
anaesthetics	herbicides	PVC
bleaches	house foundations	refrigerants
blinds	insecticides	shower boxes
carpets	lubricating oils	soap (unless made
cosmetics	mouth wash	from vegetable
detergents	non-organic flour	bases)
disinfectants	packages of food and	solvents
disposable medical	cosmetics	tap water
products	paints	toiletries
drains and guttering	paper unless TCF	toothpaste
drapes	(totally chlorine-	toys
drycleaning fluids	free)	vinyl
electrical cables	pesticides	window frames
electrical equipment	petrol	wood preservatives
flooring	the Pill	work tops

All chemical groups are dangerous and everyone is exposed to them. We breathe them, eat them, and drink them. There are nearly 50,000 different pesticides alone based on some 600 or so active ingredients, and combinations of two or three compounds at low levels can be 1,600 times more toxic than any one individual compound.

Even the interaction between the active ingredients and the 'inert' ingredients in a product can hugely exacerbate toxicity. For instance xylenes (solvents) have been linked to a variety of health problems including reduced fertility, increased cases of foetal resorption, increased incidence of cleft palate and decreased foetal weight. Zylene is often an unidentified 'inert' ingredient in chlorpyrifous products, used to spray homes for pests.

Many other OCs and toxic chemicals are used to manufacture finished products containing OCs, and millions of litres of

OC-bearing waste is dumped into coastal waters, affecting the wildlife, fish, and the rivers that often feed our water supplies.

Organochlorines are particularly worrying because they act like oestrogens, disrupting our own delicate hormonal balance by mimicking or blocking our own oestrogen action. Exposure to OCs is linked to damage of the reproductive system, including altered levels of sex hormones, miscarriages, abnormal sperm and low sperm counts, poor sperm motility, infertility, an increase in foetal deaths, stillbirths, and congenital defects, genito-urethral abnormalities, and undescended testicles.

Prenatal exposure, especially to solvents or pesticides, has been linked to foetal death, miscarriages, and low birth weight. Extensive studies in the United States indicate that women who have high exposure to chlorinated water supplies have increased incidence of foetal deaths or spontaneous abortions, and that neural tube defects were tripled. We are not just exposed to chlorine through drinking tap water. Whenever you turn on a tap, have a shower or flush the toilet you release toxins into the air.

Heavy Metals

Exposure to the following heavy metals has been linked to subfertility, miscarriage, stillbirths, premature birth, skeletal deformity, behavioural and learning problems and mental retardation.

Aluminium

Aluminium interferes with nutrient availability, especially magnesium, iron, zinc, copper, boron and phosphorus. It is found in additives and anti-caking agents in processed foods, baking powder, cookware, foil-wrapped foods, fats and acid foods, antacids, some water supplies, antiperspirants and toothpaste.

Cadmium

The main source of cadmium is tobacco. It is also found in refined flour, and in some water supplies. It is used in the manufacturing of batteries, fertilizers, paint, and television sets. Cadmium kills the cells of the testes in the male. Mothers who smoke while pregnant have significantly raised cadmium levels in the amniotic fluid and placenta, which have a negative correlation to the baby's birth weight and head circumference.

Lead

Lead is in the air, and in food grown in soil polluted by exhaust fumes. It is also found in unlined cans, which is why canned foods should not be stored in the can once opened. Cigarette smoking increases lead uptake by 25 per cent, and while in the West our water supplies are free of lead, it is a problem in some parts of the world. Much is being done to try to combat lead pollution but even low-level exposure has been linked to a number of severe irreversible health problems including infertility, miscarriage, still-births, malformed infants, and lower birth weight. In children exposure to lead can cause diminished physical and mental development, including lowered intelligence, hyperactivity and later behavioural problems.

Other Poisons

Nicotine

The smoke from tobacco contains more than 4,000 known poisons. Tobacco lowers testosterone levels in men, affects spermatogenesis, lowers sperm count and motility, and is a factor in impotency. Various studies show the number of children born with a malformation rises directly with the number of cigarettes smoked by the father per day.

If the baby has been exposed to passive smoking following birth, then he or she has an increased risk of Sudden Infant Death Syndrome (SIDS), asthma or hyperactivity occurring. In women, tobacco increases the risk of ectopic pregnancy, and is linked to a neonatal death rate that rises directly with the number of cigarettes smoked per day. This is in part caused by a damaged placenta that cannot nourish the baby or sustain a pregnancy. The placenta may haemorrhage, causing a premature birth and an underweight baby. The risk of a miscarriage is double that of a non-smoker, and premature births increase with the number of cigarettes smoked by the mother from 11 per cent for ten cigarettes per day to 33 per cent if 30 are smoked daily.

Foetal malformations are also increased. These include abnormalities of the central nervous system, minor brain damage, cleft palate and hare lip. Studies show that as the child of a smoking mother develops, growth is retarded and learning difficulties and behavioural problems can occur.

Marijuana

Marijuana causes lowered blood testosterone, lowered sperm count, impotency and diminished libido. Sperm motility is affected with an increase in abnormal sperm.

It upsets the menstrual cycle, causes labour complications, a lower birth weight, chromosomal damage, heart defects and behavioural problems in the developing child.

Alcohol

Alcohol can cause male impotence, atrophy of the testes, diminishing sperm count and motility. In the female alcohol reduces fertility by compromising egg development. It is also linked to chromosomal abnormalities in the baby.

In the pregnant woman alcohol crosses the placenta and travels through the baby's bloodstream in the same concentration as that of the mother's. Excessive alcohol consumption during pregnancy can cause foetal alcohol syndrome (FAS). Babies suffering from FAS are underweight and small at birth. Despite special postnatal care they often fail to thrive, and growth is slow. Other abnormalities include small head size, mid-facial tissue defects, limb and joint abnormalities. There is possible mental retardation and as the baby develops there may be behavioural problems or extreme nervousness.

Foetal alcohol effect (FAE) is the term given to babies whose condition is not as impaired as those suffering FAS. FAE symptoms include poor growth, lowered intelligence, and behavioural problems. In children who were followed through to adulthood, one study found that the problems exacerbated rather than lessened as they grew older.

Alcohol and all social drugs should be avoided for a minimum of six months prior to conception by both partners, and by the mother for the duration of pregnancy and lactation.

Caffeine

Men should avoid taking coffee or any drink containing caffeine as it inhibits sperm motility. Large amounts of caffeine can cause complete sperm immobilization. In women, caffeine consumption has been linked to spontaneous abortion, and babies whose mothers consume high levels of caffeine during pregnancy may suffer chromosomal abnormalities, congenital abnormalities and SIDS.

Intangibles

Radiation

Radiation causes free radical damage to the body's cells and may cause chromosomal, chemical and protein changes and destruction. In animals, non-ionizing radiation from microwaves, VDUs, lasers, radio frequency waves and television screens have been found to affect many of the body's systems adversely, including the endocrine and reproductive organs. In humans, VDU users have a higher incidence of miscarriage and stillbirths than non-users.

Microwaves can deeply penetrate the body causing a rise in temperature, and high intensity microwaves create heat strong enough to damage the cell lining of the testicles. Men exposed to microwaves have been shown to have a higher risk of fathering Down's syndrome babies.

Electromagnetic fields

Electromagnetic fields have been implicated in many areas of health. In one study women with fertility problems had more than four times the risk of their babies suffering from congenital urinary tract anomalies if they had used an electric blanket during pregnancy. The risk was greater if an electric blanket had been used during the first trimester, and increased with prolonged use of an electric blanket. If you do use an electric blanket, turn it on to warm the bed and off at the wall before getting into bed.

Heat

Heat inhibits sperm development. No links between heat and fertility problems have been found among women. However, there is evidence that hyperthermia may prevent cellular division, and adversely affect foetal growth, brain size and function. An American study shows the risk of spina bifida increases 31 times for women who take hot baths. However saunas, spas, or baths of less than six minutes' duration have not been shown to cause a problem.

We have looked here at factors relating to the body, the mind, diet, and the environment that can contribute to difficulties in conceiving. Although the detailed summary of causes of infertility may seem rather daunting, natural therapies can easily help correct some of these imbalances, and strengthen your body so that you can cope better with the environmental toxins that are impossible to escape. There is much you can do to eliminate toxins from your home and garden. For example, by eating organically you can cut your exposure to organochlorines and organophosphates by 90 per cent. The next part of the book will give you constructive help in these various aspects of your life.

Part 2: Taking Control and Giving Nature a Chance

5

Understanding the Signs of Fertility

Now that we have identified the causes, physical and otherwise, of subfertility, we can consider some straightforward, practical ways in which you can make a difference to your levels of fertility. This part of the book takes a close look at how to understand your fertility patterns so that your chances of conception will be enhanced. It gives practical advice on changes you can make to your diet, and suggests ways in which you can improve your environment at home and at work. It also provides some useful tips on how to relax, something that may seem difficult to achieve when becoming pregnant has become a significant issue in your relationship.

Because timing is such an important factor in successful conception, understanding the signs of fertility in a woman is a crucial first step towards enhancing your chances of falling pregnant. You can begin by charting your menstrual cycle and observing changes in your mucus and body temperature. If your natural health practitioner is not familiar with charting, you should make an appointment with the local Family Planning Centre. Learning to read the signs of fertility is not difficult, and can be something you are both involved in as a couple. Some have found the process has brought them much closer together and has thus reduced the stressful aspects of trying for a baby.

Nature has given us clear indicators of a woman's fertile days within each menstrual cycle. The chart on page 48 illustrates the changes in a typical 28-day cycle, and traces the release of hormones during this time. It also shows what happens to the endometrium, the egg follicle, and the cervix.

As you can see, there are several different ways of identifying your fertile days. By observing the characteristics of your mucus, noting the changes in your body temperature, and feeling the changes in your cervix, you can learn to 'read' when your body is most fertile.

Using a Chart

Some couples find it helpful to record the changes during the menstrual cycle on a chart. Charting is controversial. It is retrospective, and some experts are convinced it puts too much pressure on the couple to perform at a specific time. Others consider it is a necessity. I have treated many cases of subfertility successfully without charting, but there is no doubt as to its benefits. It is exciting to think that by charting your pattern for a few months you can recognize your fertility signs, and learn to work with your body.

If you do decide to use a chart, please never *demand* your partner perform because 'this is the moment'. Never forget to be his lover, romantic and giving. Your child will then be conceived as it should be, with love. In many cases correct timing is all that is necessary for conception to take place.

Reading Your Mucus

Your mucus is vital to conception and is fertile just before and at ovulation. Its production is governed by your hormones. If you are ovulating, but not producing fertile mucus, then the sperm are not going to be able to withstand the acidity of your vagina, or be nurtured and directed through the uterus to the fallopian tubes where fertilization takes place.

Each woman has her own mucus patterns and different factors can alter mucus characteristics. Once you have learned how to recognize your unique pattern, you will be able to differentiate between infertile and fertile mucus.

Following your period, you may not notice any mucus, or if you do it will be thick, sticky and white or cream in colour and feel dry to touch. This is known as your basic infertile pattern (BIP). Your BIP may be noticeable for approximately four days.

Over the next two days, as oestrogen levels rise, there may be a slight increase in the amount of mucus. It will still be thick and sticky, but the vulva area will feel moist.

Over the next four days approximately, the mucus becomes more profuse, watery, clear, stretchy and wet, rather like egg white. It may be translucent, milky white, or occasionally tinged with blood. This spotting is due to the effect of oestrogen on the endometrium. This wet mucus is fertile mucus. At its most fertile, mucus is known as 'Spinn' (Spinnbarkheit). It is wet and slippery, and is often described as resembling egg white. Don't worry if you do not experience this. Not all women do. Just remember 'wet' mucus is fertile mucus. The last day of fertile mucus is known as the *peak day*, and for most women it is one day after ovulation. So during these fertile days be generous with your love-making without becoming clinical. The fact you *know* this time you could make a baby should make you both all the more ardent.

Following ovulation, the change from fertile to infertile mucus can be sudden or gradual. Under the influence of progesterone the mucus reverts to being thick, opaque, and moist. For two or three days it is still semi-fertile. This is followed by approximately seven days with no mucus. Towards the end of the cycle, mucus may again be thick and opaque reducing to a watery moistness prior to the first day of menstruation.

It is important that you get to know your different mucus patterns, in particular the change from 'dry' to 'wet' mucus. Texture, colour and amount must be carefully charted until you have a clear picture of your fertility pattern – generally three to five cycles is all it takes for most to become proficient mucus readers.

There are factors that may confuse your mucus observation, such as residual ejaculate from previous intercourse, sexual excitement, nutritional deficiencies, stress, hormonal imbalances, drugs, or cervical polyps, warts, cysts or surgery. Vaginal douches, sprays or lubricants can also upset the fine pH balance of the reproductive organs and should never be used.

On the blank chart on pages 52–3 there is space for your mucus readings. Remember, you will not need to chart constantly – just until you learn to work comfortably with your body and learn to understand by observation your body's signs of fertility. It is so important to note every relevant detail, though, including incidents that may alter your mucus.

Figure 5 Changes during the menstrual cycle

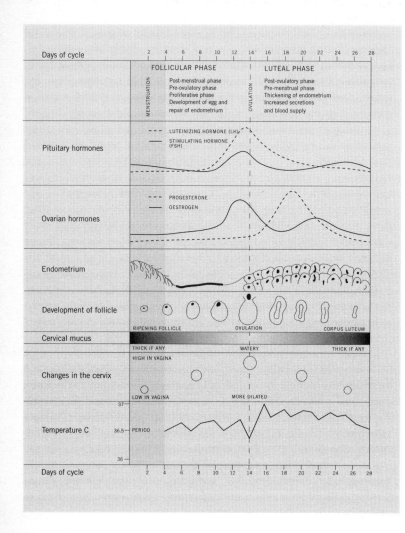

Charting Your Temperature Patterns

Another change that occurs throughout your cycle and indicates ovulation or pregnancy is your basal body temperature (BBT). When charting your temperature patterns it is important to work with Natural Family Planning, or with a natural health practitioner. If you look at the chart (page 48) you will notice a slight temperature dip as the ovum is released from the follicle. This dip is experienced only by about 30 per cent of women, so don't worry if your chart does not show it.

More important is the temperature rise or shift, which indicates ovulation took place 12 hours prior to the rise. While this is the most common pattern, there are cases when ovulation occurs up to five days prior to the rise, or up to two days following the rise. You will have your own unique pattern.

Although the temperature indicator is retrospective, at least it gives you a clear indication that you are ovulating. By observing your patterns month by month for four or five cycles you can confirm your day of ovulation.

As your mucus is semi-fertile for a short time following ovulation, you could try to conceive on the second or third temperature peak. The rise of 0.2–0.4°C may be sudden or gradual and is caused by the effect of progesterone in the blood. Towards the onset of the period the temperature falls. If you are pregnant, your temperature stays elevated.

Taking and charting your BBT is simple. A digital print-out thermometer is recommended as they are easier to read and will 'bleep' in just one minute when your temperature will be clearly recorded. This must be done first thing in the morning once you are fully awake, in bed, before *any* activity at all. Have your thermometer, chart and pencil beside the bed. If you are clever enough to read the slight temperature changes of your cycle on an older mercury thermometer you must hold it under your tongue for five full minutes. You can note the temperature on your chart when you get up.

If you wake earlier than usual, your temperature may be marginally lower. If you wake later, the temperature may be marginally higher. Temperature changes can occur with lack of sleep, shift work, travel, trauma, illness or medication such as aspirin. Just remember that no matter how your routine is interrupted, you must take your temperature daily, noting any changes that could influence your reading.

Changes in the Cervix

Cervical palpation is another means of 'reading' when your body is fertile. Many women will prefer to concentrate on observing changes in vaginal mucus and in body temperature. However, noticing changes in the cervix involves little more effort than using a tampon. When you are fertile, the cervix feels wider, wet and soft. It will be higher in the vagina. During the infertile days it is easier to feel as it is lower, hard, and may just feel like a dent rather than an opening. At the most fertile time of the month the opening of the cervix dilates slightly, making it more receptive to the passage of sperm.

Helen's story

After four years of trying for a baby and being told there was nothing wrong with me, it was suggested that I begin studying my mucus and charting my temperature as a means of discovering if I was ovulating – and to make sure we were trying to conceive when the time was right. I am 28 years of age and Gary is 34.

The first month was not very successful. I thought I noticed changes in my mucus production, and the graph looked as if a spider had walked over it. At least I noticed that my temperature did appear to go up a little after two weeks.

The second month, I became more sure my mucus was doing the right thing, and I got my graph looking quite professional. It gave me quite a thrill! The third month was easy, and the consecutive graphs showed I should have no trouble conceiving.

Our natural therapy treatments, which started at the beginning of all this charting, consisted of nutrients, and a change in diet. Three months later I became pregnant, and delivered Jos full term, all of him joyously strong and healthy.

I had to wonder what I had got myself into when I was asked to track my mucus and my temperature, but I now use these two methods as a contraceptive. I no longer need to use the charts. It's funny to be thinking of stopping babies when we had so much difficulty with Jos, but we want to enjoy him and let him have his baby years exclusively. When he is two then hopefully we will be able to have another – without any problems. I recommend these methods to any woman. It is so good to feel in control, and working together has added a special dimension to our marriage.

Date																
Description of mucus																
Day of cycle	1	2	3	4	5	6	7	8	9	10	11	12	13	14	15	16
37°C																
.9																
.8																
.7																
.6																
36.5																
.4																
.3																
.2																
.1																
36°C																
Cervix																

UNDERSTANDING THE SIGNS OF FERTILITY

17	18	19	20	21	22	23	24	25	26	27	28	29	30	31	32	33	34	35

6

Your Body and Your Food

Never before has nutrition been so vital to our general health, to our ability to conceive and carry a baby well, and to the health of the babies we deliver. Nutritional deficiencies are a major cause of fertility problems. Getting serious about nutrition means looking at your diet, and making dietary reform a major priority on your self-help list. We should try to eat food as close as possible to its natural state.

Whenever you change anything in your life, especially your diet, do it slowly. A gradual introduction of new tastes and foods will not cause a revolt in the household or upset your digestive system. However, when it comes to fertility, the more you can do to move to a natural diet, the quicker and better will be the result. If you don't like something the first time round, forget it for a while and try it again later. If your taste buds have only known refined foods, they are probably not going to take immediately to real foods.

Getting Started on Healthy Eating

Here is a list of tips to help you both move towards a wholefood diet.

- Vegetables and fruits should be fresh, not tinned or frozen. The fresher the better, and organic is best of all.
- Grains should be whole, not refined. Use brown rice, for instance, not polished white.
- Flour should be stoneground, wholemeal or unbleached. White flour and sugar should be eliminated from your pantry.
- Avoid storing fresh vegetables and fruit in the refrigerator for more than a few days, as the nutrients leach and diminish.
- Overcooking vegetables also reduces the nutrients. Try lightly steaming vegetables instead of boiling them.
- Avoid eating too many concentrated foods such as packaged fruit juices, purées and vegetable oils (except cold-pressed oils).
- You can be sure your vegetables are chemical-free if you grow your own. No matter how small your garden, it is possible to

harvest at least some of your own food. Use compost-filled pots on the balcony or patio. Try growing different varieties of lettuce, herbs, broccoli, spinach or silver beet, courgettes, beans, cucumber, or mesclun. Mesclun, a mixture of green salad leaves, can be grown all year round. It grows fast, and as you cut the tender fresh leaves off, a fresh crop appears within days.

- If you are disinclined or for some reason you cannot grow your own fruit and vegetables, buy organic. There are excellent sources of organic produce and meat all around the country.
- Avoid processed, 'junk' foods, and fast foods. These are low in nutrients, high in salt, oil and refined carbohydrates, all of which prevent many of our body pathways functioning efficiently.
- You will want to keep one or two processed foods in the pantry, but choose those with no additives and preservatives, and keep their use to a minimum.
- Never fry foods. Try browning onions in a little stock or water. The oils least damaged by heat are peanut oil, sesame oil and olive oil. If you must cook with oil, follow the old Chinese practice of placing a little water in the pan, then the food, then the oil. The natural goodness of oil is distorted through heat, so don't overheat the oil during cooking. Alternatively, add a little oil to foods just before serving.
- Completely avoid caffeine, which is found in chocolate, coffee, cola, and energy-type drinks. Alcohol must also be avoided preconceptually. Weak green tea can be taken in moderation.
- Avoid any foods that contain chemicals, preservatives, colourings, and at each meal always include something raw, such as a salad or a piece of fruit.
- Try expanding your tastes. Some foods you may not have considered; for instance, instead of butter or margarine try tahini (sesame spread), nut butters, avocado, or a fruit spread for your bread or toast. Make your own mixed wholegrain cereals to have with fruit for breakfast or as porridge in winter.
- Buy your organic wholegrain flours, nuts and seeds with a recent 'packed on . . .' date, and keep in an airtight container, preferably in the fridge. These goods are more prone than commercial varieties to rancidity as they have not been sprayed and still retain their precious oils.

FOODS THAT CAN INFLUENCE OESTROGEN

Phyto-oestrogens (plants that contain oestrogenic compounds)
Legumes including soybeans, green beans, red beans, split peas, mung beans, chick peas, peas, especially sprouts, Alfalfa, aniseed, brassicas, celery, cherry, clover, fennel, hops, sage, parsley, pumpkin, rhubarb
Wholegrains – barley, buckwheat, corn, millet, oats, rye, wheat
Oils – sesame, sunflower, linseed
Herbs – black cohosh, false unicorn root, ginseng, liquorice, passion flower, peony, red clover, sarsaparilla, wild yam

Plants and foods that promote body oestrogen
Alfalfa, aniseed, garlic, liquorice, olives, parsley, potatoes, sage
Dairy products, eggs, animal protein
Apples, cherries
Cereals

Foods that help reduce oestrogen levels of the body
Berries, citrus, dill, figs, grapes, melons, onions, pears, pineapples, squash, thyme

ACID/ALKALINE FOODS

Acid foods
Alcohol, all animal proteins, antibiotics, coffee, fried foods, grains (except oatmeal and millet, brown and wild rice), hydrogenated oils, milk products, nuts (except almonds), peas, soybeans and soy products, sugar, tea

Alkaline foods
All vegetables and fruits, almonds, lentils, molasses, soy sauce.

Neutral foods
These can be eaten often. Aubergines, beans, buckwheat, dates, eggs, fish, flaxseed oil, honey, oatmeal, organic olive oil, rice (wild and brown), turkey

Ensuring Your Daily Nutritional Needs Are Met

Protein

Protein is essential for fertility. It is found in meat, poultry, fish, eggs, milk, cheese, yoghurt, nuts, seeds, pulses, wholegrains, and in some vegetables such as mushrooms, corn, broccoli, asparagus and cauliflower. Ensure you have daily a supply of good protein, which should make up one third of your daily food intake. Many of the best-known sources of protein are from animal produce, which contain saturated fat that is far from healthy.

One of the best proteins is fish because besides being easily digested, fish contains many other important nutrients including essential fatty acids in the form of omega-3 triglycerides, and there are no saturated fats to worry about. Shellfish is also a good source of protein, but it should be harvested from waters well away from industrial wastes and sewage. You should have fish two or three times a week.

Lean meat with no fat may be taken twice weekly. When choosing meat, make sure it is lean and cut off any visible fat because this is where the toxins are stored, unless the meat is organic. Vary your intake, and use free-range organic chicken, organic eggs or cheese one day in four. Dairy products should be used minimally because of their tendency to cause allergies.

If you are vegetarian, you must know how to obtain a whole protein from your diet. You can get a complete protein by combining wholegrains such as brown rice, pot barley, buckwheat, millet, wholewheat or rye products with nuts, seeds, and pulses such as lentils, soybeans, legumes or sprouts. Always keep a supply of nuts, seeds, wheatgerm, and brewer's yeast, to add to your protein dishes.

Complex carbohydrates

Two thirds of your diet should comprise unrefined complex carbohydrates, the bulk of which should be green leafy vegetables, eaten raw when possible; other varieties of vegetables eaten raw or lightly cooked; grains; fruits; and in smaller amounts nuts and seeds, seasonings, naturally fermented vinegar, and cold-pressed oils. If you have trouble digesting raw foods, try very small amounts, gradually increasing the quantities as your digestive system becomes used to them.

Most modern diets use too many grains and cereal products. These are mainly highly refined, and we have come to regard them as staples. Even breads labelled 'high fibre' and 'multi-grain' are often highly refined. Try making your own bread with organic stone-ground flour. One or two slices are all you can manage, it's so full of body, and the taste is of real bread. There is no mystique in bread-making. I make mine as I'm getting the evening meal.

RECIPE FOR REAL BREAD

7 cups wholegrain flour (include a mix of grains)
2 teaspoons sea salt
2 tablespoons cold-pressed oil (sunflower, olive)
3 cups warm water
2 tablespoons yeast
2 tablespoons honey

Dissolve the yeast and honey in $\frac{1}{2}$ cup of the above measurement of water. When the yeast mix has doubled in size, add it to the flour with the remaining water, salt and oil. Mix together in a mixer or by hand. Place mixture in two loaf tins and leave to rise in a warm place. Bake for 35–45 minutes at 150°C.

Variations:
Add nuts, seeds, groats, sprouted seeds, wheatgerm, or bran as part of the flour quantity.

Fats and oils

First some definitions. Oils are liquid, fats are solid. The chemical term *lipids* refers to fats, oils, cholesterol, and fatty acids which are the main building blocks of fats and oils. Phospholipids comprise the membrane that surrounds and protects our cells. Linoleic acid (LA) and alpha-linoleic acids (LNA) are two essential fatty acids (EFAs) we need, but our bodies cannot make them without the right foods. Sources of LA and LNA are oils such as linseed or flaxseed, safflower, sunflower, corn, evening primrose and sesame.

There are good fats and bad fats. Most of the fats we take into our bodies in today's diet are saturated fats – the bad fats. They are found in palm or palm kernel oil and coconut oil, which are common ingredients in processed foods. They are also found in meat, eggs and in dairy products such as butter, milk and cheese.

Good fats are needed for healthy reproductive organs and adrenal glands, eyes and ears, and brain function. The right fats are also important for cell protection and as an energy store. If your body is starved of good oils, the health of any baby you give birth to can be seriously impaired. Good fats must be cold-pressed, unprocessed and fresh. They should not have been exposed to heat, light, oxygen, hydrogen or acid during their processing. As soon as oils undergo any processing to make margarine, cooking or salad oils, they are no longer healthy foods. They become just as dangerous to our bodies as saturated fats, because their chemical structure has been changed and cannot work with our bodies. Oils in their natural state are known as CIS oils. The molecules and chemicals that make up the oil are arranged in a way that enables the oil to work with and be utilized by our bodies. CIS oils are destroyed by heating, hydrogenation, bleaching, and deodorizing – processes most oils on the supermarket shelves go through. Processing converts them from CIS to trans oils.

Trans fats disrupt cellular behaviour, allowing toxic substances to enter the cell, causing abnormal functions implicated in high cholesterol, cardiovascular and degenerative diseases and cancer. If you see the words 'partially hydrogenated' or 'hydrogenated' on a label, the product contains trans oils. The more solid the product, the higher the trans fat levels.

Fish oil or omega-3 is necessary for brain function, protection against degenerative diseases and healthy reproductive organs and glands. Increase the quantity of fish in your diet, but also consider supplementation from salmon, sardines and mackerel, as it is difficult to achieve the therapeutic amount required by the body through diet alone. You may like to combine omega-3 with omega-6 (evening primrose oil). The best oils to use are sunflower, safflower, pumpkin, sesame, olive, wheatgerm, walnut, almond and rice bran. Purchase oils in small quantities in dark bottles and store in the pantry away from direct light. Use a variety of cold-pressed oils, rotating them on a day to day basis.

Seasoning

Avoid cooking with salt as it draws out moisture and essential nutrients. Experiment with herbs and spices, a little cold-pressed oil (vary your usage), apple cider or balsamic vinegar, a few drops of lemon juice, honey or seeds to bring out flavours. If necessary use a light sprinkling of herb salt once cooling is complete. Your taste buds will soon adjust and learn to enjoy the true flavours of foods.

Beverages

Replace soft drinks with diluted freshly squeezed fruit juices, herb teas which can be drunk cool, or pure water with a few sprigs of mint or lemon balm from the garden. Another pleasant drink is one teaspoon of apple cider vinegar and one teaspoon of honey in a glass of water. Use only purified water as tap water contains OCs and other poisons.

In the suggested meals that follow, some foods are recommended to be eaten twice weekly or one day in four. These food groups have a high risk of allergy, and as such should be avoided when you are trying to enhance your fertility, and during pregnancy. A baby free of allergies is happier and healthier than one who, as he or she grows, develops asthma, eczema, glue ear, or has frequent infections and sleep, behavioural and learning problems, which are just a few allergy symptoms.

Easy Meal Suggestions

If you know or suspect you have a low blood sugar problem (hypoglycaemia), then you should always have a piece of fruit before rising in the morning, a snack mid-morning and mid-afternoon, and before you go to bed. An excellent combination to take either for breakfast or dinner is brown rice and millet in the ratio 2:1 (approximately) as this can help regulate your insulin and therefore blood sugar levels. Some of the symptoms you may experience with hypoglycaemia are acute fatigue, weakness, irritability, restlessness, dizziness, and a headache if you have not eaten for a few hours or if you miss a meal.

BREAKFAST

Breakfasts are often rushed and seldom enjoyed. Try any of the suggestions below for a nutritious start to the day. If you don't have time for porridge or eggs during the week, have them at the weekend.

- A bowl of home-made muesli, made with rolled oats, rice flakes, wheatgerm, millet flakes, freshly ground linseeds, almonds, sunflower and pumpkin seeds, dried fruit, coconut thread. Add fresh fruit, organic soy or rice milk.
- Oats, rice flakes or millet porridge with organic soy or rice milk. Use a combination of grains in the porridge mix.
- Cooked brown rice, dried fruits, nuts and seeds. The rice can be prepared the night before and stored in a thermos. Just before eating, add sliced banana, a little maple syrup and organic soy milk, rice milk or diluted coconut milk.
- Cut up a pear and toss gently with cashew nuts and chopped dates.
- If you are not allergic to yoghurt add a little to your favourite fresh fruits one day in four.
- A lightly poached or boiled egg one day in four.

Have fruit with every breakfast, either fresh, dried, or in the form of freshly squeezed diluted fruit juice. With every breakfast also have a slice of wholegrain bread with honey, fruit spread, or good-quality yeast spread. Drink green or herbal tea or herbal coffee.

LUNCH

You can vary your lunches according to the season. Always try to have a piece of fresh fruit.

In winter have a home-made soup with lots of vegetables – leeks, carrots, parsnips, pulses, onion, celery, pumpkin, brown rice or barley, and fresh herbs. If you are working, soup is easily transported in a thermos, and many workplaces have cooking or heating facilities.

In summer make a large salad with green leafy vegetables such as young spinach or silver beet leaves, or finely shredded cabbage. Try Chinese cabbage, mesclun leaves, different varieties of lettuce leaves, watercress, sprouts, and herbs such as coriander, parsley, lemon thyme, mint, basil, or chives. Add colour and texture with other vegetables in season such as red cabbage, radish, peppers, cucumber, grated baby carrot or young courgette. Salads can be dressed with olive oil and apple cider vinegar, garlic, and other herbs, and a little honey. Or try a touch of soy sauce and sesame oil, fresh grated ginger, and a little curry spice.

Some additions to a salad are:

- Diced sweet potato and/or pumpkin cooked in a little water till tender, then tossed in a small amount of olive oil and a dash of curry spices with a little garlic.
- Lightly steamed beans, diced apple, pear, tiny broccoli or cauliflower florets, nuts and seeds, dried fruits.
- Banana, steamed brown rice made into a salad with tuna or salmon, basil, chives, parsley, and a chopped hard-boiled egg. Bind with dressing as for salad. Or wholegrain bread.
- Twice weekly have a baked potato in its skin.

If you rely on packed lunches, simply prepare a small container of salad, or a wholegrain sandwich packed with salad vegetables, plus dried fruit, nuts and seeds and fresh fruit.

DINNER

Your dinner can be as elaborate or simple as you care to make it. Good fresh food does not need a lot of preparation. However, the evening meal often has to be prepared when you are tired from a day's work, and it can be a bit of a drudge.

Get your partner and anyone else in the household involved in the preparation if you don't like cooking. You will find it much more enjoyable.

Start with a soup or freshly made vegetable juice. Then have each one of the following:

- A small raw salad.
- Lightly cooked vegetables (not starchy varieties), tossed together and wok steamed with garlic and herbs until just tender. Before serving add a touch of lemon juice or balsamic vinegar, a sprinkling of sesame seeds, and fresh herbs.
- Good quality protein. Rotate the form of protein over a four-day cycle: day 1, fish; day 2, lamb; day 3, a vegetarian combination or fish; day 4, chicken.

Dessert should be fruit based. Goat's milk yoghurt may be added twice weekly.

SNACKS

Between meals take plenty of liquids – pure water, fresh diluted juices, herbal teas or herbal coffee. Fresh fruit or dried fruit, nuts and seeds may be taken as snacks.

If you need something more substantial make an organic wholegrain fruit loaf or muffins. There are some good-quality whole rye crisp breads or interesting rice wafers available from the supermarkets and health shops.

Apart from maximizing your health, eating a natural wholefood diet will keep you at your ideal weight. For optimum fertility and a healthy pregnancy you should be neither under- nor overweight.

John and Caroline's story

After three years of trying to conceive, investigations showed John's sperm to have poor motility and a count of 9 million per ml. His wife Caroline was also tested and as she was not ovulating was prescribed Clomid. She had no other health problems. Because of John's sperm count and motility, they were not considered suitable for assisted conception. After eight cycles Caroline began ovulating, but there was no improvement with John's sperm. A year later they began eating organically. Eighteen months later John's sperm count had increased to 36 million and motility was good. They decided to use IVF, although technically a pregnancy could have occurred naturally. On the first natural cycle Caroline conceived and nine months later had a strong healthy daughter weighing in at just under eight pounds.

7

Improving Your Environment

Anything you can do to reduce the amount of toxins you are exposed to in your home, garden or workplace is well worthwhile. Have a close look at the following suggestions, and identify what you can do straight away without too much upheaval and reasonable cost. You can start by eliminating chemical products and using non-toxic alternatives.

Taking Action Around the Home

Minimize household cleaners, laundry detergents, bleaches and other detergents. Use only truly environmentally friendly ones. Labels can be misleading, so make sure you check the active ingredients with the manufacturer and avoid any formulated with petrochemicals and fragrances, synthetic phosphates (NTA or EDTA), optical whiteners, chlorine, synthetic surfactants, ammonia and benzene.

You can also use old-fashioned cleaning agents.

A GENERAL CLEANSER CAN BE MADE FROM
1 part white vinegar to 1 part water, or 4 tablespoons washing or baking soda dissolved in 5 cups warm water.

Check the base of the containers of any food you buy. PVC is identified by number 3 in the triangle. Don't buy it. PVC-free packaging includes:

- polyethylene terephthalate (PET) – identified by number 1 in the triangle;
- high density polyethylene (HDPE) – number 2;
- low density polyethylene (LDPE) – number 4;
- polypropylene (PP) – number 5.

If you are choosing toys for a child, look for those made from wood or other natural materials. The plastic used in many toys is often PVC.

Keeping Pests Under Control

To deter flies, keep your surfaces spotless. Clean up immediately after snacks and meals, and do not leave food uncovered on worktops. Avoid leaving surplus animal feed in your pet's feeding bowl, as it will attract flies. Try using fly swats instead of fly sprays and consider installing fly screens.

Don't use chemical flea collars on pets. If you are using direct applications to treat animals for fleas, wear gloves to apply the insecticide, and do not let children near the pet for four to six hours. A good safe product that combats dust mites and fleas is now available from pharmacists.

NATURAL FLEA TONIC	
For dogs: 2 tablespoons dolomite 2 tablespoons kelp 4 tablespoons garlic powder 4 tablespoons brewer's yeast Mix together and use 1–2 teaspoons in their food each day.	**For cats:** Mix $\frac{1}{4}$ teaspoon of garlic powder with their food each day.

Around the Garden

Seek out alternatives to insecticides, pesticides and fertilizers. Learn, instead, the basics of companion planting, or investigate the natural garden products such as garlic and pyrethrum for all garden pests, natural slug and snail bait, and natural fertilizers made from fish by-products, seaweed and enzymes.

Use citronella candles outside on patios and at barbecue time.

Building or Renovating a Home

If you are lucky enough to be building or renovating your home, ensure all your pipes, cabling and building materials do not contain PVC. They will continue to emit chlorine toxins all their life. Check that any plastic product you choose is either PE (polyethylene) or PP (polypropylene). Both of these are totally chlorine free. Alternatives to PVC are aluminium, clay or ceramic products. Any wooden product or item of furniture should not be treated with chemical toxins and should come from certified, sustainable sources.

In place of vinyl flooring and wallpapers, choose cork or ceramic tiles, uncoated wallpaper made from totally chlorine-free paper, or water-based paints and sealers. Choose carpets without latex backing, and ensure they have not been treated with stain resistance, pesticides or fungicide. If you cannot avoid these have them stored for four to five months before installation.

When choosing blinds, consider wood or bamboo, or inquire what kind of plastic the blinds are made from. Avoid plastic and synthetic curtains. Use natural fabrics for furnishings, and pure cotton bed linen rather than polyester blends.

Open windows whenever possible, especially if you have a newly built home or have done any renovations.

If you have a swimming pool, consider changing from chlorine to an ozone salt system. When buying garden furniture, choose wooden, metal or PE plastic.

Personal Hygiene and Safety

To protect yourself and your family from mosquitoes or sandflies, use natural treatments and creams. These are harmless and available in strengths suitable for babies, children and adults. Use reputable natural cosmetics, hair products, toothpaste, and vegetable-based chemical-free soaps and washing liquids.

Tap water is heavily chlorinated, so use a water purifier or a water filter, or have spring water delivered in bulk to your door.

Only use microwaves when absolutely necessary. Use non-PVC cooking containers and never cook commercial meals or frozen meals in their packaging. Do not open the door while the oven is on, and have the microwave checked regularly for leaks.

When watching television, make sure you sit at least six feet or a few metres away from the screen.

To avoid exposure to radiation, heat your electric blanket before going to bed, and pull the plug from the socket before getting into bed. Avoid having any electrical appliance such as a clock radio close to your head when sleeping.

Some wet-weather gear is made from PVC. Choose either leather, PP or PE plastic, or a waxed fabric instead.

Avoid long hot baths, spas and saunas.
Don't smoke.

In the Workplace

If you work with visual display units, ensure you have regular periods working at other jobs, and use protective shields that reduce the rays. Some modern screens are anti-radiation.

Encourage your employer to use natural commercial-strength cleaners.

Bring in a few plants. Not only will these brighten your environment, but they will give off oxygen, take up carbon dioxide and remove some of the toxins from the closed environment.

Have a break out of the office at lunchtime. Go for a walk, especially if you have a park nearby or are close to the sea.

You can work on these aspects of your lifestyle gradually, changing your cleaning and personal hygiene products at a reasonable cost as you renew your supplies. Have a look around your home to see what, if anything, you can change in the house without incurring too much upheaval and unreasonable cost. Anything you can do to take even a small amount of toxic load off the body is going to be beneficial to you and your baby. For maximum protection ensure you take a daily antioxidant formula – vitamins A, C, E and zinc. These will help protect your cells from destruction by environmental toxins.

8

Looking After Your Body and Your Mind

Maintaining a balanced lifestyle means paying attention to rest, recreation and relaxation as well as your diet and environment. The 'three Rs' are interdependent. Relaxation will come easily if you exercise regularly and can enjoy good, deep sleep every night. Spending quality time together as a couple just having fun is especially important if you are feeling the strain of trying to have a baby. Consciously make time for each other, and your friends – and never pass up the opportunity to have a good laugh.

Exercise

There are many benefits to regular exercise. As well as toning the muscles and improving your strength and flexibility, it helps slow the ageing process, improves concentration, and helps in dealing with stress, depression and anxiety. Exercise is important for good overall, and therefore hormonal, health. If you are not used to exercising regularly, try to fit in 20–30 minutes daily, or at least three 30-minute sessions weekly. Some people prefer the discipline of going to the gym regularly, or joining a yoga or aerobics class. However, if classes are not for you, try to incorporate a good brisk walk into your daily routine. Take your partner or a friend with you. Or go swimming a few mornings a week. Commit to making regular exercise part of your routine.

Yoga is not only an excellent form of exercise, it also teaches you deep relaxation. It tones the muscles through stretching, activates the glands, and quietens the mind. The classical Hatha form of yoga is a perfect, yet gentle form of exercise. Well learnt, with a little bit of discipline, it can be done in the privacy of your own home, and once it becomes part of your daily routine you will find you miss it when you don't practise it. Rebounding or trampolining is an excellent aerobic exercise that can also be done at home and, like yoga well learnt, increases muscle tone and circulation, tones the endocrine glands and lymphatics, and relieves congestion.

You can count good bustling housework, gardening, or mowing the lawns as part of your exercise time. Over-exercising is as bad as too little exercise, so just remember the old adage: everything in moderation.

Getting a Good Night's Sleep

We all know a tired body does not perform well sexually, so make sure you both get sufficient, good-quality sleep. If you have trouble getting to sleep or staying asleep, your therapist will be able to help you, whichever modality you choose. However, if sleep does elude you, you might like to try some of the following ideas.

- Incorporate more exercise into your daily routine, especially if you have a sedentary job or lifestyle. Choose a form of exercise you truly like, rather than forcing yourself into an exercise programme you are uncomfortable with.
- Avoid having a heavy meal at night.
- Reduce your intake of refined foods, especially sugar, caffeine and food additives. These are not conducive to good sleep.
- Do not go to bed too early or too late, and do not read in bed. Equate your bedroom and your bed with sleep.
- Never try too hard to go to sleep. Often the harder you chase sleep, the more elusive it becomes.
- Relax or meditate before bedtime.
- Have a warm bath with the luxury of essential oils. Try basil, camphor, camomile, lavender, marjoram, neroli, rose, sandalwood, or ylang ylang.
- Herbal teas can also help you relax before bedtime. Try verbena, camomile, lemon balm, valerian, lime flowers, skullcap, hops, passionflower.
- Reduce your alcohol intake. Alcohol can destroy your store of magnesium and the B vitamins, which are all so important for relaxing the nervous system, normal brain activity and sleep rhythms.
- Supplements of calcium, magnesium, potassium, zinc, vitamin B and vitamin C with bioflavinoids will encourage relaxation and sleep.
- If you have an emotional concern or worry, seek help from a professional counsellor.

- If you have any physical discomfort such as digestive problems, joint pain, nasal congestion or restless legs, seek help from a health professional.

Relaxation and Visualization

Rest or sleep is different from being able to relax the body completely, and being able to truly relax is in turn conducive to good healthy sleep. With practice you will be able to use the technique given in the panel below to help you relax. For those of you who have done yoga, this will be a familiar style of exercise. Initially you will probably need somebody to quietly and slowly take you through the steps, or you could try making a tape recording of the steps in the exercise. Choose your time well, when you know you will not be interrupted for at least 15 to 20 minutes.

RELAXATION AND VISUALIZATION EXERCISE

Lie on the floor with your legs slightly apart, and arms out a little from your side, palms up.

Close your eyes.

Tighten your toes by curling them up . . . and relax them. Pull on the ankles . . . and relax. Pull on your knees . . . and relax. Tighten your abdomen . . . and relax. Pull on your chest muscles . . . and relax. Tighten your throat . . . and relax. Pull the shoulders forward, press them back . . . and relax. Stretch your arms down to the end of your fingertips, curl your fingers tight . . . and relax. Lick the lips, drop the jaw a little and keep it in that relaxed position. Screw up the eyes . . . and relax. Run your mind over the body, seeking out any parts that are still tense and using this same technique of tightening and letting go, relax your body completely.

Be aware of the rhythm of your breathing without controlling or regulating it. You will feel so relaxed that you feel heavy, like a great log that has been lying in the warm sand for many years. As you become aware of your breathing, slowly the heaviness gives way to a lightness. You feel so light, it is like lying on a cloud (or on sand, or a riverbed . . . invent your own place of 'retreat' and use the same one every time you relax). You feel happy, tranquil, and totally in control of your mind and body.

Your mind is free of incoming thoughts. If they waft in, let them waft out again. Imagine they are part of a television screen you have no interest in. If any thoughts are troubling you, let them go. Imagine them leaving the body on the outward breath.

On the inward breath, take in a golden glow of lightness, filling the mind, entering every cell, healing, strengthening. Hold your thoughts on each reproductive part of your body. Imagine your ovaries producing perfect eggs, your tubes, healthy, functioning well and open, ready to receive your partner's sperm and transport your fertilized egg, your uterus, full, ripe and healthy, ready to hold and nurture your baby.

Now slowly stretch back to reality. Return yourself to the everyday world, knowing your body is becoming healthier by the week, your mind more relaxed, your attitude more positive.

Part 3: Natural Remedies and Other Treatments

9

Choosing a Natural Therapist

Although the practical steps outlined in Part 2 can help improve fertility, many couples find that natural remedies and other treatments greatly enhance their chances of conceiving. In this section we look at a wide range of treatments that require the help of a practitioner. We look at mineral, vitamin and herbal supplements, and other treatments such as homoeopathy, osteopathy, massage, aromatherapy, and sex or couple counselling. There are also self-help directions for many common ailments related to fertility. However, in some situations self-help is inappropriate. If in doubt, seek professional advice from a qualified health practitioner.

Subfertility is seldom, if ever, the result of just one problem, but a combination of factors that must be clinically assessed. While there are many ways in which you can help improve your own fertility, a natural health practitioner must be part of your self-help plan. Some treatments detailed in this part of the book, such as acupuncture, by their very nature necessitate a visit to a practitioner. However, naturopathy is really an extension of your self-help programme and is not as visit-oriented as other forms of treatment. Your biochemical requirements must be clinically assessed by a practitioner, but the dietary and lifestyle part of the treatment is carried out by you every day.

Whichever therapy you choose, your practitioner will assess your problem by examining you as an individual who has a unique pattern of biochemistry, energy flows, and therefore symptoms. In your first consultation you may be asked questions that do not seem to relate directly to your problem. Your practitioner will also be interested in how you relate to your environment. Questions about how you react to noise, heat, cold, dampness, foods and drinks will enable your practitioner to prescribe with total accuracy. These types of questions are combined with different diagnostic techniques specific to the therapy you have chosen, to determine your treatment protocol.

Each therapy discussed in this part of the book has been practised for hundreds or thousands of years, and yet their success has only begun to be viewed scientifically in recent years. Each is based on a strong philosophy, and each is safe.

If you are in doubt about who to go to, ask among your friends. Your health professionals should also be able to make good recommendations. (Also refer to the list of helpful addresses at the back of the book.) Never feel shy about phoning and talking to different therapists. It is vitally important to have a good rapport with the person you will be working with. Most therapists are only too pleased to discuss how they can help you. The first consultation can be as much your assessment of the practitioner as theirs of you.

Self-help can only help so far. For example, the vitamin and mineral supplements given in this part of the book will certainly enhance fertility, in a general sense. However, if you have your individual needs precisely assessed by a naturopath, then your treatment will be all the more effective and give faster positive results. Your formula will be put together with a minimum of tablets using a combination of nutrients that is balanced according to your needs. As your health improves, you may need to be reassessed because of changes in your body. However, you should not need to visit a naturopath more than once every four weeks initially, and then once every eight weeks, but this is dependent on each case.

A naturopath will also help isolate and address masked food allergies, and will provide helpful hints and general assistance in eliminating allergies. Naturopaths follow safe, scientific protocols when prescribing herbal remedies. They will help you overcome problems of chemicals and toxins in your particular environment, and will guide you towards reasonably priced alternatives. If you have been exposed to chemicals, then your supplements will be adjusted to help you overcome the effects of exposure.

Couples invariably want to know how long natural treatments will take to work. Realistically it is difficult to give timeframes of success. Pregnancies can occur quickly once treatment has started especially when nutrition is used as the 'ground work' therapy. However, regardless of the therapy you choose, it is important to balance the nutritional levels of the body in order to achieve a trouble-free pregnancy and a healthy baby. Most practitioners therefore suggest waiting four months before trying for a baby. Despite your sense of urgency, it is worth the wait.

No matter what type of natural therapy you choose, it is essential that you are able to work comfortably with your practitioner. Whichever modality you prefer, whether acupuncture, homoeopathy, osteopathy or naturopathy, your practitioner will be able to co-ordinate other treatment modalities they think will benefit your particular case. Above all, you will need a therapist who will support you by being empathetic as well as instrumental in helping you both fulfil your desire to have a healthy baby.

Susan's story

There was no apparent reason for my infertility. I had had several attempts at IVF and GIFT but had not conceived, and though my husband wanted me to try assisted conception once more, I couldn't. I felt terrible on the drugs, and hated the actual procedure. It was in desperation that I turned to a naturopath. I also had bouts of acne, and occasional migraines and constipation. These quickly got better on the programme, and it was explained that these problems were all caused by the same biochemical deficiency that was part of my fertility problem.

I was asked not to try for a pregnancy for four months. I avoided my allergens, improved my diet, took my supplements, relaxed more, got in a bit of exercise, and five months later I was pregnant. I delivered a daughter when I was 36, and 18 months later became pregnant again and delivered another healthy daughter.

10

Minerals

Fertility is not just about conceiving a baby. It is about producing a healthy baby. If we remember that the sperm and egg take about 100 days to develop we can see why it is so important to supplement for at least four months prior to trying to conceive. Many practitioners prefer a six-month period, but this may be asking a lot when a couple is so desirous of making a baby. Some researchers are now saying that it is the health of both parents in those four months prior to conception that sets the standard of health of the baby – not just for infancy but his or her entire life. What an exciting gift to be able to give your baby.

The most important aspect of supplementation is getting the balance right, for deficiencies never occur singly as each has an interaction with others.

Minerals act as catalysts for the utilization of all other nutrients. They enter thousands of biochemical pathways, and without minerals no vitamin can function properly. Daily mineral losses through bile, sweat, urine and faeces are 7000 mg. This must be replaced on a daily basis. We certainly cannot do this on a modern diet. As you read through the following pages, note how much of each nutrient is lost through minimal processing, and try to come to terms with this in a collective sense. It doesn't leave us with a lot, does it?

There are some 56 minerals present in the human body. Of these the body needs calcium, chlorine, magnesium, phosphorus, potassium, sodium and sulphate in bigger amounts. These minerals are known as macronutrients. Other minerals needed in smaller amounts are known as micronutrients. Minerals that are of particular importance to fertility are potassium phosphate, magnesium phosphate, zinc, iron, selenium, silica, manganese, and iodine. The combination of potassium phosphate and magnesium phosphate is important for nerve and muscular health, the relaxation of muscles and organs, and hormonal activity. Muscle tone improves and depression is lifted with these minerals. Combined with sodium phosphate, these minerals also help regulate the acid–alkaline balance of the body and stabilize the heart.

MINERALS	
Mineral	**Where you can find it**
Calcium	Kelp and other seaweeds, salmon and sardines with bones, hazelnuts, almonds, brazil nuts, green leafy vegetables, tofu, ground sesame seeds, raisins, molasses
Chromium	Brewer's yeast, liver (organic), molasses, shrimp, wholewheat, asparagus, egg yolk, oysters, mushrooms, nuts, prunes
Copper	Almonds, mushrooms, oysters, lamb, pork, prunes, sunflower seeds, wholegrains
Iodine	Fish, oysters, kelp, iodized salt, lima beans, mushrooms, sunflower seeds, onions, dark green leafy vegetables
Iron	Liver, lean meat, oysters, green leafy vegetables, molasses, dried fruits, wholegrains and pulses
Magnesium	Unmilled or stoneground wholegrains, wheatgerm, corn, dark green vegetables, parsnips, sunflower and sesame seeds, almonds and cashew nuts, apples, figs, seafood, brewer's yeast, molasses
Manganese	Wholegrains, green leafy vegetables, kelp, olives, liver, nuts, seeds, corn, pineapple, egg yolk
Phosphorus	Almonds, cashew nuts, sesame seeds, tuna, chicken, eggs, garlic, salmon, chickpeas
Potassium	Wholegrains, all vegetables, especially leafy green varieties, mint, potato skins, bananas, citrus, dried fruits, pulses, sunflower seeds, almonds, cashews, pecan nuts
Selenium	Brewer's yeast, garlic, wheatgerm, bran, wholegrains, sesame seeds, and meat, provided the animals are fed on produce grown in selenium-rich soil

Silica	Found in the fibrous parts of vegetables and grains, especially root vegetables, barley and oats
Sodium	Seafood, meat including liver, celery, kelp, vegetables and fruit
Zinc	Pumpkin and sunflower seeds, oysters, herring, meats including liver and kidney, brewer's yeast, wholegrains, wheatgerm

Calcium

Calcium phosphate is one of the prime needs for good cell development, and therefore growth. It forms the basis of the skeleton, is important for nerve and muscle function, cardiac and blood health, and the secretion of many hormones. It activates enzymes and aids regulation of nutrient use. Calcium uptake in the body is reduced by dietary fat, oxalic acid, and phytic acid. You must therefore ensure all your grains are soaked or cooked before eating. Other foods affecting calcium balance are citrus, potatoes, tomatoes, peppers, aubergine, sugar, honey, too much protein, salt, vinegar, wine, alcohol and dairy products. This mineral is used to treat amenorrhoea, dysmenorrhoea, and for painful erections in men. Calcium phosphate should be taken with magnesium and vitamins A, C, D, E.

Chromium

Chromium is part of what is known as the GTF (Glucose Tolerant Factor), along with proteins (amino acids) and niacin. It is important for insulin efficiency and the regulation and metabolism of glucose, preventing hypoglycaemia and diabetes. It is also thought to be involved with the synthesis of protein, fatty acids and cholesterol – and cholesterol is needed to make hormones. Even the slightest deficiency can have serious effects, particularly when there are other deficiencies that have not been treated. The foetus needs lots of chromium, and so pregnancy can cause a deficiency, a symptom of which can be nausea. About 45 per cent of chromium is lost in food refining and processing.

Copper

Copper can cause fertility problems if the body has too much or too little. If there is an imbalance, it is usually too much copper. A blood or hair test will indicate your levels.

Iodine

Iodine is a mineral that influences hormone balance. It is important for a healthy thyroid and general physical and mental development. A deficiency can cause fatigue, low libido, tumours of the pituitary gland, high blood cholesterol and weight gain, all of which could contribute to a state of subfertility. A deficiency in the pregnant mother can lead to cretinism in the baby. Like most nutrients, if given in excess it can cause serious health problems. Refined foods are generally devoid of iodine.

Iron

Iron should be given in the non-toxic phosphate form, with calcium, selenium, B complex vitamins and vitamin C and beta-carotene. If you have difficulty absorbing iron, you could be deficient in potassium sulphate or vitamin C. White sugar and white flour in the diet, and an imbalance of gastric acidity can also hamper absorption. Iron should never be given alone as it can cause other deficiencies – particularly of zinc, chromium, manganese, selenium and cobalt.

Magnesium

Magnesium phosphate acts as a catalyst in more than 300 biological reactions, and in all reactions involving energy production within the cells themselves. Magnesium is necessary for the maintenance of the nervous system, and for protein and DNA synthesis.

It must be part of any treatment where there is anxiety, depression or tension – and as there is always an emotional aspect to fertility problems, the combination of potassium phosphate and magnesium phosphate is often used in a treatment programme. Ninety per cent of magnesium is lost during milling of grains.

MINERALS

Manganese

Manganese should be given with zinc because of its importance in maintaining efficient sex hormone production. It is also needed for good skeletal development, nerve and brain function, enzyme activity, lipid metabolism and a good healthy milk supply. Between 80 and 90 per cent of manganese is lost through milling.

Phosphorus

Phosphorus works together with calcium, magnesium, potassium and sodium. It is found in every cell of the body, and is therefore involved in almost all chemical reactions, nutrient synthesis, energy cell division and reproduction, is important for the glands, muscles, nerves, kidneys, and in helping to maintain the correct alkaline–acid balance.

Potassium

Potassium is involved with nearly 50 enzyme pathways, and, with phosphorus, influences cell replication and division. It also enhances brain oxygenation. With calcium it regulates neuromuscular activity. Potassium is leached from food during processing.

Selenium

Selenium can be an important consideration as there is a gross deficiency of this mineral in certain soils. Animal studies link this deficiency with infertility. It is also a powerful antioxidant and detoxification agent, especially for toxic metals such as cadmium. Selenium works better when taken with vitamin E. Approximately 50 per cent of selenium is lost during milling.

Silica

Silica is also often deficient in the body. Its role is structural. It is necessary for strong muscles, tendons, bones, cell walls, clean healthy arteries, the development of the placenta, calcium usage, and helps in the detoxification of heavy metals. Silica is lost through food refining.

Sodium

Sodium receives a lot of bad press, mainly because we have overloaded our systems with too much sodium chloride or common salt. The mineral sodium is vitally important because of its relationship with potassium, and if given in the phosphate form will help maintain the correct acid/alkaline balance in the body, an important factor in digestion and vaginal acidity. It stabilizes blood pressure, negates the accumulated effects of common salt, and acts as a catalyst for the efficient absorption of other minerals. It is important for nerve and adrenal function.

Sodium sulphate has a beneficial effect on the liver, aids detoxification processes, and maintains the correct balance of body fluids.

Zinc

Zinc, like magnesium, is one of the most widespread mineral deficiencies in the Western world. Zinc is essential for the functioning of more than 200 enzymes, DNA and RNA metabolism, and efficient male and female hormonal activity. It is one of the most important factors in the development and functioning of reproductive organs, the development of the prostate, seminal vesicles and testes, and for normal healthy sperm and sperm counts. Many a case of impotency has been reversed with zinc. A deficiency of zinc compromises the body's immunity, and an optimum immune system is paramount to protect both mother and baby. Stretch marks, now often seen in girls approaching puberty, and white flecks on the fingernails are signs of a zinc deficiency. A zinc deficiency worsens with pregnancy and can result in post-natal depression and poor lactation. For the developing infant, problems can involve retarded sexual and mental development and learning difficulties. Zinc absorption is inhibited by calcium and iron, and should therefore be taken at different times. Eighty per cent of zinc is lost during milling of flour.

You can see from the various interactions of minerals how complex it can be to strike the right balance for each individual person. Doses for minerals depend on the kind of supplements used, and the results of your personal assessment. It is rare for a naturopath to prescribe large doses of any nutrient, but they do work with therapeutic doses, and elemental amounts of nutrients rather than the chemical form most often noted on the labels. For example, if you buy a calcium gluconate supplement, you will receive only 9 per cent of the total milligram weight as elemental calcium. Some forms contain as little as 1–2 per cent of the mineral itself.

The following is a list of minerals and general dosages that will certainly help improve your fertility. However, for optimum benefit your deficiencies should be assessed clinically or with a hair test from a reliable laboratory that will give not only deficiencies but also excess levels. You should not need separate supplements for each of these nutrients: look for combinations. For instance, zinc is often formulated with magnesium, manganese, and other synergistic factors. Selenium is usually part of a good antioxidant formula. If you cannot match the given amounts perfectly, do not worry. The suggested dosages are a guide only and well within the safe dose range.

The individual cells of our bodies are a collection of minerals and water. Mineral deficiency is the most common cause of many health problems. Once you have achieved the right balance of minerals in your body, you have laid a solid foundation for the success of any other treatment you and your practitioner want to employ.

MINERAL SUPPLEMENTS FOR MALE FERTILITY	
Zinc	50 mg
Manganese	40 mg
Magnesium	300 mg
Selenium	75–200 mcg
Chromium	100–500 mcg
Potassium (usually in the chloride form)	260 mg

MINERAL SUPPLEMENTS FOR FEMALE FERTILITY	
Calcium	500–800 mg
Magnesium	half the amount of calcium; however a deficiency could indicate your need for a 1:1 dose
Zinc	50 mg
Manganese	10 mg
Iron phosphate	15 mg
Selenium	150–200 mcg
Chromium	500 mcg
Potassium	200–300 mg

11

Vitamins

Vitamins are organic substances found in plants and animals. Without them we could not live, and yet, with a few exceptions, we cannot synthesize vitamins ourselves. We should ideally obtain them from organic foods, but when there are deficiencies in our diet and in the food we buy, we have to rely on good-quality supplements to develop therapeutic doses.

Vitamins, like minerals, are dependent on many interacting factors. To use vitamin C as an example, a supplement may provide vitamin C only in the form of ascorbic acid. No fruit gives us just ascorbic acid, but a complex of nutrients such as flavonoids, and other vitamins in minute amounts, along with minerals and enzymes. A good vitamin C product would therefore contain a variety of ascorbates and flavonoids, and the base should contain a combination of acerola cherries, citrus and/or rosehips to give you all the other nutrient factors in tiny doses. This ensures all the co-factors of the central nutrient (in this case vitamin C) in the supplement are present, and makes the supplement work better. You will get maximum value from your supplements if you take them with a good wholefood diet.

What Vitamins Do for Fertility

As we have said so often – any supplement taken in higher doses should be under the supervision of a health practitioner. As for minerals, your vitamin intake should be individually assessed, according to your specific needs.

Although we will be concentrating on fertility in this section, the systems and parts of the body that are strongly dependent on each particular vitamin will also be mentioned where appropriate. The whole body has to be healthy for the reproductive system to be healthy. Vitamins are important for making a healthy baby. Many tissues are dependent on vitamins, but no vitamin can work without minerals.

FOOD SOURCES OF VITAMINS

All fresh fruit and vegetables contain a small amount of most nutrients. Vitamins, like minerals, incur huge losses with storage and processing.

Vitamin	Rich food sources
Vitamin A	Dark green leafy vegetables, broccoli, red peppers, carrots, tomatoes, apricots, cod-liver and fish oils, kidneys, liver, egg yolk, dairy products (not skim milk)
Thiamine (Vitamin B_1)	Brewer's yeast, wheatgerm, wholegrains, yeast, molasses, liver
Riboflavin (Vitamin B_2)	Avocado, sprouts, broccoli, currants, liver, tongue, kidneys, eggs, brewer's yeast, wholegrain cereals, milk
Niacin, nicotinamide, nicotinic acid (Vitamin B_3)	Lean meats, poultry, fish, almonds, peanuts, brewer's yeast, wheatgerm, desiccated liver
Pantothenic acid (Vitamin B_5)	Brewer's yeast, egg yolks, wheatgerm, wholegrains, kidney and liver, legumes, avocado, green leafy vegetables, mushrooms, salmon
Pyridoxine (Vitamin B_6)	Meat including offal, salmon, tuna, brewer's yeast, wholegrains, molasses, legumes
Folic acid (Vitamin B_9)	Green leafy vegetables, liver, brewer's yeast, lentils, eggs
Cyanocobalamin (Vitamin B_{12})	Animal protein, especially liver, kidney, fish and dairy products. Soy, kelp, and some types of brewer's yeast contain small amounts of B_{12}
Vitamin C	Citrus, and all fresh fruits and vegetables, rosehips
Vitamin D	Cod-liver oil. Sunlight is also a source

Vitamin E	Cold-pressed, unrefined oils, nuts, seeds, wheatgerm, wholegrains, avocado, green leafy vegetables, egg yolk
Essential fatty acids (EFAs) (Vitamin F)	Fish, especially salmon, mackerel, sardines, cod, evening primrose oil, safflower oil, sunflower oil, wheatgerm oil, corn oils, linseeds, sesame seeds, nuts, soybeans. Smaller amounts are found in dark green leafy vegetables, seaweed, and broccoli

Vitamin A (retinol, retinoic acid, beta-carotene)

Vitamin A is a fat-soluble nutrient requiring fats and minerals for proper absorption. Carotene (beta-carotene is the most active) is changed in the intestine to vitamin A with the help of zinc. Vitamin A is essential for normal growth and general reproductive health. Tissues dependent on vitamin A are the mucous membranes that line the uterus, the fallopian tubes, digestive and respiratory tracts, the eyes, skin, hair, blood and bones. It is necessary for the conversion of cholesterol to oestrogen and male androgens. It has strong antioxidant properties and should be given with other antioxidants, vitamins C and E, zinc and selenium. A deficiency can cause degeneration of the gonads, failure to conceive, or a tendency to miscarry. If the woman is seriously deficient in vitamin A, the baby could be born without eyes or with a cleft palate. Pregnancy and lactation increase the need for vitamin A. However, doses in excess of 10,000 iu daily can also result in birth defects. Beta-carotene is a good safe form to take. So too is cod-liver oil, which also gives you vitamin D and a small amount of precious essential fatty acids. Toxicity is generally in doses in excess of 26,000 iu per day for two years or more.

Vitamin B

Vitamin B should always be taken as a complex, that is, as a combination of single vitamin substances. If there is a gross deficiency of an individual B vitamin, it should be given with a tablet containing the full complex as an individual B vitamin taken alone can create other B deficiencies. The complex is water-soluble. The B group of vitamins is concerned with energy and good digestion. Vitamin B keeps the gastrointestinal tract healthy, and thus aids elimination. It is necessary for the health of the nervous system (helping to combat stress), the cardiac system, the mouth, tongue, skin, eyes, and liver. It also aids immunity.

The need for the complex as a whole increases with pregnancy and deficiencies are implicated in hormonal imbalances, especially low progesterone, the hormone that holds a pregnancy. Pregnancy problems and malformation of the baby can be severe with just a slight deficiency of any one aspect of this complex.

The above general benefits of the B complex are applicable to each aspect of the individual B vitamins.

Vitamin B_1 (thiamine) is important for energy production, growth and learning ability, the central and peripheral nervous system, muscles, cardiovascular system, thyroid, digestion, enzyme function. The need of B_1 increases with pregnancy, particularly if your diet includes refined foods, sugar, caffeine drinks and alcohol, if you exercise excessively, or if you have only recently come off the Pill. A deficiency has been associated with infertility, miscarriage, stillbirths and low birth weight, retarded growth and Down's syndrome. Toxicity is rare.

Vitamin B_2 (riboflavin) is critical for a healthy pregnancy in that it affects hormone levels and follicle development. If you have a B_2 deficiency, then infertility, stillbirths, resorption or a severe malformation of the foetus can occur. Vitamin B_2 is important for liver health, skin, hair, and eyes, and maintenance of various tissues of the body. There is no known toxicity for B_2.

Vitamin B_3 (niacin, nicotinamide, nicotinic acid) is important for brain metabolism, sex hormone and lipid synthesis. Niacin is vital to general growth and for the circulation.

Vitamin B_5 (pantothenic acid) is required by every cell in the body. It is important for adrenal health, steroid hormone production, lipid, protein, carbohydrate metabolism and vitamin absorption. It helps protect against stress, fatigue and excessive radiation, and reduces the adverse effects of some antibiotics.

Vitamin B_6 (pyridoxine) is important in infertility as it influences progesterone levels. The need increases with pregnancy and lactation. It is necessary for the mental and physical growth of the foetus. It is also needed for the metabolism of essential fatty acids and consequently prostaglandin activity, the proper functioning of RNA and

DNA, antibody and red blood cell production. It helps maintain the balance of sodium and potassium in the body, thus regulating body fluids and normal functioning of the nerves and muscles. B_6 is needed for B_{12} absorption and efficient usage of zinc, magnesium, and manganese.

Vitamin B_9 (folic acid) is needed for good sperm and egg production. If you have been on the Pill, your folic acid will have been depleted. Prior to conception and in the very early stages of pregnancy, folic acid is important for healthy chromosomes, cell differentiation, organ development of the embryo, and for the prevention of neural tube defects. An excessive intake of folic acid can mask a B_{12} deficiency. It is best to take these two together – and with a full vitamin B complex and EFAs.

Vitamin B_{12} (cobalamin, cyanocobalamin) is the only vitamin that contains a mineral, cobalt, which is vital to longevity. It aids the synthesis of RNA and DNA and blood cells, helps the efficient functioning of iron and vitamin A, and is needed for the metabolism of fats, proteins and carbohydrates. It is important for the maintenance of epithelial cells, gut mucosa, bone marrow and body lipids (fat and fat-like substances) and growth. The vitamin is difficult to absorb, needing calcium, a healthy thyroid and the presence of hydrochloric acid. If you are vegetarian, ensure you have sunflower seeds and other sprouted seeds, as these, along with peanuts, allow B_{12} to be synthesized in the gut. Use peanuts with caution as they are commonly linked with allergies. B_{12} should always be taken with folic acid, as they work together.

A vitamin B complex may also contain biotin, choline, inositol, para-aminobenzoic acid (PABA). These aspects have similar benefits to the body as the main B factors, and any good B complex will contain them in a balanced proportion.

Vitamin C (ascorbic acid)

Vitamin C maintains collagen, the 'cement' of the body, and without healthy collagen the entire body can disintegrate. It is important for the nervous system, brain, maintenance of cell membranes, blood cell formation, digestion, sugar metabolism, absorption of other nutrients, the immunity and healing. It is a powerful antioxidant, diuretic, detoxifier, and anti-stress agent. Vitamin C has a strong link with fertility and is needed in a rich supply throughout a pregnancy. It facilitates the production of sex and other hormones and regulates cholesterol metabolism. The ovaries, adrenal, pituitary and thyroid glands are all dependent on ongoing supplies for efficient functioning. In the male, it is important for good sperm motility. If the expectant mother has a good ongoing supply of vitamin C, the baby is more likely to be healthy. A good vitamin C supplement should contain co-factors, bioflavonoids, sometimes known as vitamin P. Given the levels of toxic exposure we are all subjected to, most people do not take sufficient vitamin C. The need for the vitamin increases if you have been a smoker, have had symptoms of toxin exposure, allergies, or have been on the Pill.

Vitamin D (D₃ – cholecalciferol) (D₂ – ergocalciferol)

Vitamin D is a fat-soluble nutrient and is needed to metabolize calcium and phosphate for healthy bones and teeth. This interaction with calcium and phosphate also makes it important for a healthy skin, nervous system, heart, and normal blood clotting. Vitamin D is absorbed from the ultraviolet light of the sun on our skin. The best food source is cod-liver oil, as vitamin D should be given with vitamin A, and this oil gives the two nutrients in the right ratio. The need for vitamin D is increased with pregnancy and lactation, especially if you are vegetarian, are deprived of sunlight, or if you suffer from colon problems such as ulcerative colitis or Crohn's disease, as this nutrient aids the synthesis of enzymes in the mucous membranes necessary for calcium absorption. Like other vitamins, D is also a complex. Vitamin D_2 is a synthetic vitamin not found in nature but added to foods such as milk or used in some multi-vitamins. While it is similar to D_3, which is made by the action of sunlight on our skin, it has a subtly different biochemical structure and has been implicated in problems involving calcium metabolism. In foetal development, a deficiency of vitamin D is associated with bone deformities of jaw, palate and skull, which may impair brain development. Deficiencies are also associated with retarded growth, soft teeth and bones. Eustachian tube function may be inefficient, leading to middle ear infections.

Vitamin E (tocopherol)

Vitamin E is another complex of substances. Known as tocopherol, this vitamin is hugely important to our reproductive organs, as it regulates the synthesis of sex hormones, and enhances both male and female fertility. It helps maintain a healthy pregnancy, so should be taken throughout and during lactation. A severe deficiency in the male can cause permanent damage to the testes and consequent sterility. As part of the antioxidant group of nutrients, it protects our body's cells against pollution, oxygen, the sun, and ageing. Other nutrients and saturated fatty acids and even our own hormones are protected from oxidation, which would otherwise result in free radicals that cause damage at cell level. It is also an effective healing agent internally if taken post-operatively, and if applied externally helps to prevent scar tissue. Old scars can sometimes be 'melted' by this vitamin. Vitamin E stabilizes cell membranes. It is vital for the overall health of the vascular system, improves blood flow and prevents blood clots forming. It protects against anaemia, kidney and liver damage, and prostate enlargement. Vitamin E is sensitive to heat, light and alkalinity. The Pill and mineral oils prevent vitamin E absorption.

Vitamin F (essential fatty acids)

Essential fatty acids (EFAs) are vital to our overall health. Without a good supply of these nutrients the body cannot synthesize hormone-like substances known as prostaglandins, essential for the health of every cell, moment by moment regulating our mental and physiological activity and a healthy blood supply. EFAs nourish nerve cells and mucous membranes, aid efficient insulin use, combat inflammation, and regulate cholesterol use. The nutrients are important for the production of adrenal, thyroid, and sex hormones, and for interactions with other nutrients aiding the synthesis of vitamin A, enzymes, and calcium absorption (along with vitamin D).

Essential fatty acids are greatly depleted in a modern diet. Refined foods, processed foods, saturated animal fat, cooking oils (other than cold-pressed), margarine, spreads, some breads, cakes, biscuits, fries, processed snack foods, chips, frostings, desserts, ice-cream, and alcohol all inhibit the synthesis of these precious nutrients. A good supply is necessary throughout pregnancy and during lactation for a milk supply that is EFA-rich, for this is so very important for the baby's continuing health. A well-balanced antioxidant formula, that is vitamins A, C, E, zinc and selenium, should be taken with EFA supplements. To obtain a well-rounded balance of EFAs, a combined fish oil and evening primrose oil supplement can be taken. Vitamin E

needs to be increased when taking EFAs, and some supplements
already have this added.

A Word on Enzymes

Throughout this discussion on nutrients, enzymes have often been
referred to. Enzymes are present in every cell of our body, and are
constantly required to ensure the smooth running of our bodies.
Moment by moment, millions of biochemical reactions occur to keep
us alive. Enzymes are catalysts and each is specific to a certain
reaction. They speed up biochemical reactions that would otherwise
take much longer. Enzymes comprise two parts: one a protein
molecule, the other a coenzyme. They are also found in natural raw
foods.

The following is a list of vitamins beneficial to reproductive
function. The suggested amounts given below are daily doses.

VITAMINS FOR MALE FERTILITY	
Vitamin	**Dose**
Vitamin A	6 mg (in the beta-carotene form) Converts to approximately 10,000 iu vitamin A
Vitamin C	1000–6000 mg in divided doses (1000–2000 mg three times daily)
Vitamin E	400–1200 iu in divided doses (200 iu twice daily or 400 iu up to three times daily) Check with your health professional if you suffer from high blood pressure
Vitamin B complex	Not less than 50 mg of B_1, B_2, B_3, B_5, and B_6 daily
Essential fatty acids	500–3000 mg from fish oil and/or evening primrose oil in divided doses (500 or 1000 mg up to three times daily)

Other supplements that could be taken to enhance male fertility are amino acids. L-carnitine (300–500 mg three times daily) and L-arginine (1000 mg three times daily) have been found in some studies to increase sperm count and improve motility. As these are more expensive supplements, try minerals and vitamins first. Don't use arginine if there is a history of herpes infections as this could exacerbate the condition unless lysine, which is also helpful in increasing sperm motility, is given as well.

VITAMINS FOR FEMALE FERTILITY	
Vitamin	**Dose**
Beta-carotene	6 mg (this converts to just under 10,000 iu of vitamin A, which is a safe dose for pregnancy, as facial and genital deformities may occur in a baby if conceived while the mother is on high doses)
Vitamin C	1000–6000 mg in divided doses (1000 mg taken one to three times daily or 2000 mg taken three times daily)
Vitamin E	400–1200 iu in divided doses (200 iu twice daily or 400 iu up to three times daily. Check with your health practitioner if you have high blood pressure)
Vitamin B complex	Not less than 50 mg of B_1, B_2, B_3, B_5, and B_6
Folic acid	800 mcg daily
Essential fatty acids	1000–3000 mg in divided doses (1000 mg up to three times daily)

12
Herbs

Herbs have been used to heal since antiquity. The names of herbs such as squaw vine, birthwort, motherwort, and crampbark reveal the important role they have played in restoring, regulating, and aiding reproductive health. Many modern drugs have their origins in herbs. More than 20 per cent of drugs have been taken or isolated from plants. However, once a constituent is isolated and refined or synthesized to become a 'drug', it can produce unwanted side effects and has lost the true therapeutic value and safety factor provided by the plant's complex chemistry.

The main constituents that give plants their therapeutic value are alkaloids, glycosides, tannins, bitters, mucilages, volatile oils and trace minerals. But it is the complex composition of the plant's chemistry that gives the restorative, healing effects to our body's systems and organs. Just as each plant is complex, so too are the interactions of the different herbs that go to make up each formula.

Chinese herbal preparations are available generally in powder or pill form. The formulae are carefully balanced and often thousands of years old and are matched to your needs as diagnosed according to the principles of traditional Chinese medicine. Herbs can also be given as a decoction. For instance, Chinese herbs are often given in a dried form, carefully measured to give the balance of nutrients for your particular needs. These herbs are then boiled for a specified time, then strained and the liquid taken in specified doses. Chinese herbal medicine is only available through a qualified practitioner.

Western herbs also have histories going back thousands of years, and although there are preparations available in tablet or capsule form, most medical herbalists prefer to work with liquid extracts, so that a prescription of several herbs may be formulated according to the exact requirements of each patient. While Western herbs are becoming easier to purchase from your health shop or pharmacist, herbal prescriptions are more effective than single herbs. It is the knowledge of combining herbs that is the basis of good herbal practice and responsible for its effectiveness.

WOMEN'S HERBS AND THEIR ACTIONS ON THE BODY		
Herb group	**What they do**	**Some herbs in this group**
Adaptogens	Balance and normalize the reproductive system.	Dong quai, false unicorn root, vitex, blue cohosh, and liferoot
Astringents	Strengthen the surface membranes of the organs and check excessive bleeding or discharge.	Bethroot, periwinkle, golden seal, shepherd's purse, wild indigo
Emmenagogues	Contain hormonal compounds that have a direct influence on the uterus and normalize the menstrual cycle. These should not be used during pregnancy.	Blue cohosh, squaw vine, false unicorn root, yarrow, rue
Alteratives	Stimulate the natural elimination processes of the body working through the lymphatics, kidney, skin and digestive tract, thus relieving congestion of the reproductive organs.	Cleavers, nettles, red clover, burdock, blue flag
Nervines	Relax or stimulate and restore nerve tissue and function and so normalize and strengthen reproductive tissue.	Crampbark, avena, valerian, damiana, skullcap, squaw vine

94

Demulcents	Heal and restore the tissues of the reproductive system, so are of great benefit for inflammation, irritation and infections.	Uva-ursi and marshmallow
Antimicrobials	Used when treating infections and to enhance immunity.	Wild indigo, uva-ursi, buchu, echinacea

MEN'S HERBS AND THEIR ACTIONS ON THE BODY		
Herb group	**What they do**	**Some herbs in this group**
Adaptogens	Strengthen and heal male reproductive systems.	Siberian ginseng, damiana, saw palmetto
Alteratives	Encourage efficient elimination of lymphatics, kidney, digestion and skin, remove congestion.	Blue flag, cleavers, poke root
Antimicrobials	Enhance resistance to reproductive system infections.	Uva-ursi, buchu, echinacea, wild indigo
Circulatory enhancers	Increase blood and nutrient flow to reproductive organs, aid elimination of stagnant fluids and toxins.	Cayenne, prickly ash, ginkgo, sarsaparilla
Nervines	Relax or stimulate nerve tissue and function.	Avena, damiana, siberian ginseng, gotu kola

Herbal medicine must be prescribed by a qualified medical herbalist. However, if you wish to enhance your overall and therefore your reproductive health, you can make a herb tea with organic raspberry leaves, red clover and nettles, and take it for four months prior to trying for a conception. A few drops of dong quai can be added to this tea. Neither dong quai nor the tea should be used during pregnancy. Raspberry leaf should only be used in the last trimester of pregnancy as it tones the uterus, thus facilitating an easier birth.

WESTERN HERBS TO AVOID DURING PREGNANCY		
Aloes, angelica, autumn crocus	Feverfew, false unicorn	peppermint (in high doses avoid if hypertensive)
Barberry, betony, black cohosh, bloodroot, blue cohosh, broom, bryonia, buckthorn	Greater celandine, golden seal	Rhubarb root, rue
	Hellebore	Sage, southernwood, squaw vine, senna (in high doses)
Celery seed, colchicum, costmary, cassia	Juniper	
	Liquorice (if you experience oedema or are inclined to hypertension)	Tansy, thuja, thyme
Dong quai (although a Chinese herb, it has been used for some time in Western herbal remedies)	Mistletoe, mugwort, male fern, mandrake	Wormwood
	Parsley (medicinal doses), pennyroyal, poke root,	Yarrow

CHINESE HERB COMBINATIONS FOR MALES AND FEMALES	
Combinations for women	Bupleurum and peony Bupleurum and dong quai Peony and liquorice Dong quai and evodia Dong quai and peony
Combinations for men	Anemarrhena phellodendron and rehmannia Bupleurum and zhi shi Ginseng nutritive Lotus seed, rehmannia six

ESSENTIAL OILS TO BE AVOIDED IN PREGNANCY
Basil, calamus, hyssop, marjoram, myrrh, pennyroyal, sage, thyme, wintergreen

CHINESE FORMULAE OR COMBINATIONS TO AVOID DURING PREGNANCY		
Apricot seed and linum	Clematis and stephania	Major bupleurum
Bupleurum and dragon bone	Coptis and rhubarb	Minor rhubarb
Cardamom and fennel	Linum and rhubarb	Persica and rhubarb
Cimicifuga	Magnolia and hoelen	Dong quai and peony
Cinnamon and hoelen	Magnolia and ginger	

While the above lists of Western and Chinese herbs should be avoided during pregnancy, some of these herbs are very likely to be used in a formula to enhance your fertility. Your herbalist will use a safe dose and a specific treatment timeframe.

Some of the main Chinese herbs for enhancing female fertility are dong quai, peony, cnidium, rehmannia, cornus, dioscorea, alisma, hoelen, moutan, gardenia, atractylodes, bupleurum, ginger, liquorice, evodia, ginseng, cinnamon, gelatin, pinellia, ophiopogon, schizandra.

> *Herbs for enhancing male fertility are phellodendron, rehmannia, cornus, dioscorea, alisma, moutan, hoelen, anemarrhena, ginseng, peony, atractylodes, cinnamon, astragalus, citrus, polygala, liquorice, lotus seed, ophiopogon, scute, lycium bark, schizandra.*
>
> *As for Western medicine, formulations will be according to your symptoms.*

Herbs are an important aspect of fertility treatment and, when used with dietary changes, prescribed supplements and other necessary treatments, fertility should be enhanced. Medical science has expressed great interest in herbs and as individual herbs come under scientific scrutiny, the research provides evidence of the action of the herbal actives (therapeutic compounds). It is the combination and precise dosage of herbs that make each formula so effective, which is why professional help is necessary.

13

Naturopathic Treatments for Specific Problems

One of the reasons for the success of natural therapies is that each case is assessed and treated individually. The following treatments should be viewed as a general guide only. You may wish to refer back to Chapter 3, which explains the specific causes of fertility problems. The way you present with your particular case may indicate nutrients and treatments that differ from those noted here. Your needs will determine which specific minerals or nutrients should be given. It is important to remember that just as a deficiency of a nutrient can cause fertility or pregnancy problems, so too, in some cases, can mega-doses. Practitioners prescribe well within the safe dose range.

Herbal remedies have also been given; however, the formula your herbalist prescribes for you may differ from the lists below. Some of these herbs should not be used when trying to conceive or during pregnancy. Herbal medicine should always remain the domain of qualified practitioners. No specific dosages have been given below as dosage depends on the herbal preparations used. Acupuncture, homoeopathy and osteopathy will also help most of the female and male conditions mentioned.

Do not be put off by the long lists. For most of the conditions given you will probably only need a minimum of the different protocols noted here. Practitioners vary in their treatment. I prefer a minimal approach, with a mineral formula, usually made up of three supplements, vitamins, again in combination tablets, and then if necessary a herbal formula. Dietary reform must be part of every treatment programme.

General Hormone Balancing in a Female

Minerals Magnesium phosphate, potassium phosphate (or chloride), calcium phosphate (or fluoride), silica, iron phosphate, sodium phosphate, zinc (25–50 mg), manganese (4 mg), selenium (150–200 mcg).

Vitamins Essential fatty acids (1000–3000 mg), beta-carotene (no more than 6 mg, which converts to just under 10,000 iu vitamin A),

B complex (with no less than 50 mg of main B vitamins, folic acid (800–900 mcg), and maybe 400 mcg of B_{12}).

Herbs   False unicorn root, blue cohosh, vitex, motherwort, bethroot, wild yam, liquorice, black horehound, calendula.

Essential oils   Geranium, rose, melissa. Others that may be indicated are clary, basil, lavender, marjoram, peppermint, rosemary.

Adhesions

Minerals   Potassium chloride, iron phosphate, magnesium phosphate, silica, calcium phosphate and calcium fluoride, sodium salt.

Vitamins   To prevent adhesions occurring after surgery, a good antioxidant formula should be taken which includes vitamin A (6 mg), vitamin C (1000–6000 mg or more), vitamin E (200 iu) and zinc (50 mg). These are excellent healing nutrients. Also take extra vitamin E (1000–3000 iu) for one to two months, reducing to a maintenance dose which should be continued for at least three months. The dosage should be monitored by your practitioner, although 400 iu is considered a basic safe dose. Higher doses of vitamin C and K may be required in some cases. Vitamin E may enhance anticoagulant therapy, so it should not be taken in doses above 200 iu by people on warfarin. If you have high blood pressure, your practitioner should be consulted on dosage.

Herbs   False unicorn root, golden seal, echinacea, calendula.

Amenorrhoea (lack of periods)

Minerals   Potassium phosphate (or chloride), magnesium phosphate, silica, calcium fluoride (or phosphate), sodium salt, zinc (25–50 mg).

Vitamins   B complex containing not less than 50 mg of the main B vitamins.

Herbs   Unicorn root, blue cohosh, mugwort, motherwort, ginger.

Essential oils   Camomile, clary, fennel, hyssop, juniper, myrrh.

Blocked Fallopian Tubes

Most cases require surgical intervention. If the condition is minimal, it may be treated naturally. In some cases recurrence of the problem can be prevented and natural treatment can improve recovery of the tube tissue following surgery.

Minerals   Magnesium phosphate, calcium phosphate, calcium fluoride, potassium chloride, iron phosphate, a sodium salt, silica, zinc (50 mg).

Vitamins   Beta-carotene (6 mg), vitamin C (3000–6000 mg), vitamin E (400–3000 iu).

Herbs   As for pelvic inflammatory disease, herbs will only be of use for this condition if they are used in an effective dose range. May include wild yam, golden seal, echinacea, calendula, crampbark, false unicorn root.

Cervical and Mucus Problems

Minerals   Mineral therapy benefits these problems faster than any other modality in my experience. For mucus that is too acidic or hostile to your partner's sperm, the minerals used would depend on your specific symptoms, but would always include sodium phosphate, silica, calcium phosphate (or fluoride), magnesium phosphate, with a potassium salt. You can purchase pH sticks from your pharmacy to check your treatment progress. For hostile mucus you should also use condoms for three months during which time you should follow a full nutritional programme. After this time, your first unprotected intercourse should take place just prior to ovulation. If you have undergone any cervical treatment or surgery, treat with minerals: potassium chloride, iron phosphate, silica, calcium fluoride, sodium phosphate, calcium phosphate, magnesium phosphate, zinc (50 mg).

Vitamins   Vitamin A (beta-carotene 6 mg), vitamin C (3000–6000 mg), vitamin E (400–3000 iu), vitamin B complex (with 50 mg of main B vitamins), folic acid (800 mcg). A good unperfumed vitamin E cream can be applied locally.

Herbs   Calendula, false unicorn root, golden seal. For poor mucus production: false unicorn root, vitex, saw palmetto, golden seal, bayberry.

Dietary reform   You should avoid allergens completely and your diet should contain two thirds alkaline to one third acid foods.

Dysmenorrhoea (difficult or painful periods)

Minerals   For acute symptoms: magnesium phosphate, calcium phosphate, zinc (50 mg). Other minerals must be assessed.

Herbs   Blue cohosh, crampbark, wild yam.

Essential oils   Camomile, marjoram, clary, lavender, rosemary (contra-indicated with heavy bleeding). Work with gentle massage to the lower back and/or abdomen.

Elevated Scrotal Temperature

For lifestyle and nutritional help see Chapters 6, 7, and 8.

Endometriosis

Minerals   Potassium sulphate or chloride, magnesium phosphate, silica, calcium phosphate and/or fluoride, iron phosphate, sodium salt, zinc (50 mg).

Vitamins   Beta-carotene (6 mg), B complex (50 mg of main B vitamins), vitamin C (3000 mg), vitamin E (240–400 iu daily), essential fatty acids (1000–3000 mg).

Herbs   Vitex, wild yam, golden seal, crampbark, black cohosh, red clover, dandelion, marigold, yarrow, buchu, ginger. Astragalus 8 formula should be considered if immunity is low.

Dietary reform   Should include alkaline foods – two parts to one of acid foods.

Fibroids

Treatment is similar to that of endometriosis, which is also caused by high oestrogen levels.

Minerals   As for endometriosis.

Vitamins   Beta-carotene (6 mg), vitamin C (3000 mg), vitamin E (200 iu).

Herbs   Vitex, periwinkle, bethroot, thuja, poke root, red clover, cleavers.

Impotence or Erectile Dysfunction

Minerals   Potassium phosphate, magnesium phosphate, silica, sodium phosphate, zinc (50–100 mg), selenium (100–200 mcg).

Vitamins   Vitamin E (100–750 iu), vitamin B complex (with 50 mg of main B vitamins), vitamin C (1000–3000 mg).

Herbs   Ginkgo, siberian ginseng, avena, saw palmetto, damiana, lesser periwinkle.

Essential oils   Sandalwood, clary sage, jasmine, rose, ylang ylang.

If necessary seek help from a sex therapist. (See Chapter 18.)

Male Infertility and Impotency

Minerals   Zinc (50 mg), potassium phosphate, magnesium phosphate, iron phosphate, silica, calcium fluoride, sodium phosphate, selenium (150 mcg).

Vitamins See page 89.

Herbs Damiana, avena, saw palmetto, siberian ginseng.

Essential oils Clary sage, jasmine, rose, ylang ylang, sandalwood.

Menorrhagia (heavy bleeding during periods)

Minerals Potassium chloride, iron phosphate, magnesium phosphate. Other minerals to complete the prescription must be assessed.

Herbs Bethroot, shepherd's purse, greater periwinkle, cranesbill.

Essential oils Cypress, rose.

Miscarriage

A full nutritional programme is necessary here for a minimum of four months prior to trying again for a conception.

Minerals Zinc, calcium phosphate, magnesium phosphate, potassium phosphate, silica and calcium fluoride, sodium salt.

Vitamins Vitamin A (beta-carotene 6 mg), B complex (with 50 mg of main B vitamins), vitamin C (3000–6000 mg), vitamin E (400 iu), essential fatty acids (1000–3000 mg).

Herbs Wild yam, squaw vine, false unicorn root, raspberry leaf, vitex. To aid recovery after miscarriage: bethroot, true unicorn root, blue cohosh, avena, gotu kola.

Oligomenorrhoea (irregular periods)

Follow the same remedies as for amenorrhoea.

Pelvic Inflammatory Disease

Antibiotics must be taken, but the following natural therapies can be used concurrently.

Minerals Potassium chloride, iron phosphate, potassium sulphate, magnesium phosphate, zinc (50 mg). Other minerals will depend on whether you are in an acute, sub-acute, or chronic phase.

Vitamins Beta-carotene (6 mg), vitamin C (6000–7000 mg), vitamin

E (250–3000 iu depending on the phase of the condition).

Herbs Will only be of use for this condition if they are taken in an effective dose range and may include wild yam, golden seal, echinacea, calendula, crampbark, false unicorn root.

Polycystic Ovary Disease/Ovarian Cysts

Minerals Potassium chloride, iron phosphate, silica, calcium fluoride, magnesium phosphate sodium salt.

Vitamins B complex (with not less than 50 mg of each main B vitamin), vitamin C (3000 mg), vitamin E (400–500 iu).

Herbs Vitex, false unicorn root, figwort, poke root, thuja, red clover. While small cysts respond quite quickly to natural treatment, PCOD can be difficult and take some months to treat.

Sexually Transmitted Disease

You *must* have this medically diagnosed and take antibiotics. Treatment can be supported with natural remedies.

Minerals Potassium sulphate or calcium sulphate, potassium chloride, iron phosphate, magnesium phosphate, sodium phosphate, zinc (50 mg).

Vitamins Beta-carotene (12 mg to give approximately 20 mg vitamin A), vitamin C (to tolerance level), vitamin E (400 iu).

Herbs Barberry, oregon grape, echinacea, poke root, or astragalus 8 formula. Local applications of providone iodine can be used.

Varicoceles

Surgery may be necessary.

Minerals Silica, calcium fluoride, potassium chloride, magnesium phosphate, iron phosphate, sodium salt.

Vitamins Vitamin A (beta-carotene 6 mg), vitamin C with bioflavonoids (3000–6000 mg), vitamin E (250–1000 iu).

Herbs Horse chestnut, limeflowers, stone root, witch hazel. Apply locally marigold, stone root, horse chestnut, either as a cream or solution.

Hydrotherapy is also helpful.

Chinese Formulae for Enhancing Fertility

There are many Chinese formulae, some of which may be used for both female and male infertility, well suited to Western use (see pages 97–8).

Mineral Therapy

The following table gives examples of clinical prescriptions of minerals in daily doses. These differ in form from those available in pharmacies and health shops (see pages 82–3). As they are more biologically active than other forms, doses also differ.

RECOMMENDED MINERAL DOSES			
Magnesium phosphate	65 mg × 4	Calcium sulphate	8 mg × 3
Potassium sulphate	33 mg × 4	Calcium fluoride	8 mg × 3
Potassium phosphate	33 mg × 4	Iron phosphate	15 mg × 3 or 4
Potassium chloride	65 mg × 4	Silica	33 mg × 3
Calcium phosphate	130 mg × 4	Sodium phosphate	260 mg × 3
		Sodium sulphate	195 mg × 3

14

Acupuncture

Like naturopathy, acupuncture also focuses on restoring the body to its natural balance. Originating in China more than two thousand years ago, it is one of the oldest therapies known. Acupuncture uses fine sterile needles inserted into the skin at specific points along a series of pathways, known as channels or meridians, to re-establish the energy flow, also known as the vital force or chi, which for a variety of factors can easily be disrupted and cause health problems.

The philosophy of Chinese traditional medicine is that chi is a universal energy surrounding and pervading everything, and there is a constant interchange between body chi and environmental chi. Thus, there is a concept of good and bad chi – just as there is good and bad food. Provided the body chi is strong and harmonized, the system can defend itself from harmful external chi. However, if the body chi is weakened or out of harmony, then an imbalance and ill health results.

There are 12 major pairs of meridians. Each major meridian is related to our nerves, blood vessels and body fluids, and passes through the major organs. They are connected by cross channels so all organs and tissues have access to the constant flow or movement of chi. While the cross channels can be used for carrying excess chi from one meridian to a deficient meridian, the influences of one on the other must always be perfectly balanced for optimum health.

Chi can be affected by a variety of lifestyle factors such as the stress and tension of modern lifestyles, poor nutrition, climate, lack of exercise and rest, posture, scar tissue, or emotions such as worry, anxiety, grief, frustration, depression and even joy. These factors can bring about lowered vitality and lead to fertility problems, among other symptoms.

When you visit an acupuncturist, a case history is taken. Your lifestyle habits and your likes and dislikes are noted. The acupuncturist will study the colour of the tongue, skin, facial expression and observe the patient's general demeanour and tone of voice. Diagnosis also involves palpation of the 12 wrist pulses. It is these pulses that reflect the condition of the 12 major meridians and the associated organ. Through this the acupuncturist can identify the patterns of disharmony and chi stasis.

Tongue diagnosis is exacting. The tongue is examined for colour, condition and the colour of the tongue coating. Abnormal colours are classified as pale, red, purplish-red or purple. A pale tongue may reveal a deficiency such as iron. A dry tongue may indicate disruption of the body fluids. A purple tongue often indicates circulatory problems and a stagnation of chi. The colour and condition of the coat is indicative of specific states – insufficiencies or excesses within the different organs.

By listening to your problems and how you relate to them and the environment, the acupuncturist forms a point prescription that will balance energy and normalize health and organ function. In the case of conception difficulties, sometimes it can be as simple as ridding the body of built-up stress and tension by helping to relax the central nervous system. Or the problem may lie within disharmonies of the uterus and other organs, because of lack of circulation of blood and energy to the reproductive organs.

To function well, the uterus relies on a constant supply of chi and blood. Two channels that feed the uterus are the chong (vitality) and ren (responsibility/conception), vessels which originate from the kidneys. If the kidneys are deficient, infertility or habitual miscarriage may result. Disharmony of the heart, liver and spleen can also affect fertility, for blood is governed by the heart, stored by the liver, and controlled by the spleen, so there is a close relationship between these organs, especially the liver, and the uterus. If there is liver dysfunction there may be menstrual problems. If blood is insufficient, the uterus will be starved and amenorrhoea may result. If there is too much heat in the liver, the blood flow may be too great and menorrhagia may result.

Liver chi stagnation can cause irregular periods, and if there is liver-blood deficiency, periods will be scanty or non-existent.

The above are just some of the patterns that can affect your fertility. The point prescription used during your treatments will enhance the flow of blood and energy through the lower abdomen. Once the meridians are clear, the cycle is regulated by balancing organ function and hormones.

Acupuncture can also help raise sperm counts, as in men kidney energy is closely related to sperm production, and the stagnation of liver energy will cause poor sperm motility.

If you are nervous about the thought of needles being inserted into the body, the fine needles are quite painless, except perhaps for a radiating feeling of numbness on insertion. This is known as the 'needling' sensation or radiation. The feeling is not unpleasant, and should be considered a good sign, because it indicates the chi is flowing and your energy increasing. Generally just four to six needles, bi-laterally, are used, not hundreds as some think. Moxa (a soothing, warming herb) may be used in conjunction with the needles, sending a comforting warm glow into the meridian. Chinese herbs may also be prescribed to be taken while undergoing the treatment.

Treatments are relaxing, and in fertility cases are usually scheduled according to the four phases of the menstrual cycle: pre-menstrual, ovulation, menstrual, post-menstrual.

Jill's story

Jill was 32 and had miscarried three weeks prior to her appointment. She was still bleeding, had no energy, and suffered from headaches. Other symptoms were thrush, genital herpes, occasional bleeding gums and loose stools. She had been unable to conceive for nine years and in the last year had experienced a family death, which had left her severely depressed.

Her periods had never been regular, and she had a long (27–37 day) cycle.

Her treatment harmonized the liver, strengthened the spleen energy, and consequently the 'vessels' known as ren and chong mo that help regulate the cycle and enable a conception to take place. If these vessels are weak, and conception does occur, a miscarriage is likely.

After a course of 12 acupuncture treatments over eight months Jill conceived and gave birth to a full-term, healthy daughter. This was followed by two more successful pregnancies.

Christa's story

Christa (30) was a high achiever with pressure to succeed in a tough business environment. She and her husband had been trying to achieve a pregnancy for two years. Christa's was a case of tension causing the subfertile state. Her treatment simply enabled her to relax and conception took place six weeks later. A healthy daughter was delivered full term.

Natalie and Joseph's story

At 25 Natalie's IUD was removed with considerable difficulty as it had caused an infection. Not long afterwards her periods became horrendously painful and were accompanied by bleeding from the bowel. Endometriosis was diagnosed and surgery performed to remove the endometrium. Twelve months of male hormone treatment followed to suppress her periods.

While Natalie was undergoing treatment, Joseph also started investigations with the aim of overcoming their infertility. He had a low sperm count, and after 12 months of treatment, including surgery, there was no change in his condition.

Natalie had a laparoscopy, which showed intense scarring after the hormone treatment. She and Joseph were told they would never conceive. A second opinion was sought, and they were told they would have no chance with an IVF programme. It would be a waste of money even trying.

While Natalie was coming to terms with a child-free life, Joseph found it very difficult. He suffered a nervous breakdown with headaches, tension, and uncontrollable weeping. Psychological treatment did no good. Then he tried acupuncture, and as Natalie had to drive Joseph to his treatments, she began having sessions herself, to see if she could overcome her period problems. After two years of twice weekly treatments, the first of her two children were born. She was 34, and had been infertile for 12 years.

15
Osteopathy

Osteopathy is a hands-on or manual branch of medicine. Some people find it surprising that it has a role in fertility problems. The osteopath views health problems from a holistic perspective. Since female tubal and hormonal disorders and male gonadal disorders contribute to 90 per cent of subfertility cases, then 90 per cent of cases can potentially be helped by this therapy.

After an initial assessment involving both partners, the practitioner will explain what he or she considers may be hindering fertility and what can be done to help increase the chances of conception. Prior to the commencement of treatment, laboratory tests may be necessary. Certainly a sperm count will be required if one has not already been done.

An osteopathic treatment will correct seven aspects of function that will help enable the reproductive organs to work normally.

1 *Circulation*   Good circulation of blood to and from the organs, particularly the ovaries, testes, and uterus, is vital. In some cases circulation to the pituitary gland may need to be addressed.

2 *Neurology*   All the reproductive organs have two nerve supplies that affect their function. If the activity in these nerves is increased or decreased then the organs will not be able to do their job. For example, the uterus is a muscle. It contracts during a woman's period and at childbirth. If the nerve supply to it is abnormal its tone will also be abnormal and this will affect fertility.

3 *Lymphatic circulation*   A reduction in fluid drainage from an organ by the lymphatic system results in congestion. This reduces the removal of wastes from the organ, resulting in abnormal function.

4 *Visceral (organs)*   The reproductive organs, especially the uterus and fallopian tubes, are made of muscle and ligament-like tissue. Like any muscles and ligaments, they are subject to twists and strains that affect their function.

5 *Hormonal*   This area is principally the domain of the cranial

osteopath who will ensure the pituitary gland is able to work correctly and regulate the hormonal cycle appropriately.

6 *Structural* The female reproductive organs are held in place in the pelvis by a series of ligaments that come from the walls of the pelvis (ilia), sacrum and pubic bone. Any structural asymmetry of the pelvis will cause an increase in tension in these ligaments, transmitting strain to the organs. The blood and lymphatic vessels are transferred to the organs via the ligaments. Therefore any increase in the tension of the ligaments decreases the circulation to the organs, resulting in disease.

In the male, these vessels reach the testis via a ligamentous tunnel in the abdominal wall. This is a common location for problems to arise, reducing the circulation to the testis and thus their ability to produce viable sperm.

7 *Psychological* While psychology is not the principal domain of the osteopath, any good physician must recognize the important role it plays in fertility. Stress must be managed to optimize fertility, especially if the primary cause of the stress is the fertility issue and the strain it places on the relationship between the couple.

The osteopathic approach to the problem of fertility is complex. The osteopath breaks down the problem into components and addresses each specifically. The practice of osteopathy involves much more than massage and manipulating backs. A diverse range of gentle techniques is employed, mostly to the organs themselves, to restore normal function and hence normal fertility.

Catherine's story

Catherine (28) sought help four years after an ectopic pregnancy and subsequent surgery, during which the right fallopian tube was removed. She had not conceived since then, and had during this time developed chronic constipation.

The initial assessment indicated adhesions where the right fallopian tube was removed. Contracture of this scar tissue had dragged the uterus to the right and it was twisted on the cervix. This resulted in a sharp angle where the left tube and uterus meet, and increased tension through the left tube and surrounding ligament. The tension also affected the colon, hence the constipation.

Catherine had six treatments over two months, during which the constipation resolved itself, and she conceived five weeks later. A trouble-free pregnancy resulted in a full-term, healthy son.

Neil's story

Neil's sperm count put him in the 'sterile' category. On assessment, it was found that Neil's main problem was the poor functioning of the nerve that controlled the circulation to the testes. There was also tension in the spermatic cord pulling the testes up towards the body where the temperature was too warm. His erections were impeded, and further affected by 'performance anxiety', especially if he felt he had to have intercourse on his wife's fertile days. But ten treatments over a six-month period resulted in his wife's conceiving four months later. She delivered a healthy full-term baby.

16
Homoeopathy

Homoeopathy is a complex branch of medicine. Remedies work on the principle that 'like cures like', that is, a substance that causes a disease or disease-like symptoms in healthy people can also act as a remedy for the disease, if given in a smaller dose. For example, an insect sting causes pain and swelling, so a medicine made from bee venom may treat a condition like arthritis which has pain and swelling similar to that of the bee sting. In the case of subfertility, if the fallopian tubes are blocked from the effects of a chlamydia infection, a homoeopathic medicine made from the chlamydia organisms can cause the tube obstruction to reduce substantially or completely.

A skilled professional homoeopath is able to prescribe from the huge range of medicines, choosing one to match the condition to be treated with symptoms that have been created experimentally and recorded over hundreds of years. Sometimes these symptoms are the only things felt by the patient. Sometimes they are hormone levels which can only be detected with laboratory help.

When you visit a homoeopath, a full case history is taken and you will be asked a lot of questions about your problem. The practitioner builds up a complete picture of the problem, and is able to match this to the remedy best suited to you.

Faye's story

At 37 Faye consulted a homoeopath for treatment of genital warts and painful menstruation. She was prescribed sabina, made from a kind of juniper, with the warning it might increase her fertility. Faye laughed and said she had used no contraception for 18 years and the warning was unnecessary. She conceived the month after her first pain-free period for years, and yes, the warts disappeared.

Robyn's story

Robyn had tests to determine the cause of her infertility. Both her fallopian tubes were blocked. Instead of expensive surgery, it was suggested Robyn consult a homoeopath. On hearing of a history of pelvic inflammatory disease (probably chlamydia) the homoeopath prescribed chlamydia nosode, and two months after thiosinaminum, a medicine made from a chemical derived from the mustard plant which dissolves some kinds of scars. Robyn became pregnant within a few weeks.

Amanda's story

Amanda consulted an infertility clinic and tests revealed an abnormally low level of follicle stimulating hormone. She was given a medicine made from FSH. She became pregnant the next time she ovulated.

Simone's story

Simone was unable to become pregnant despite no abnormality being found in her or her partner. The homoeopath was told that after intercourse a discharge was observed as if she expelled the semen. She had tried lying for hours with her lower back propped up with pillows and her legs elevated but that did no good. The homoeopath prescribed Natrum carbonicum, a description of which reads, 'for the discharge of mucus from the vagina after coitus (causing sterility)'. This medicine was prescribed in the 30c potency three times daily for five days around the time Simone was ovulating. After three months, she became pregnant.

Nathalie's story

Nathalie felt that she seemed to be allergic to her partner's semen – not only did she expel it, she also felt scalded internally for about ten hours after intercourse. She was given antifungal cream by her doctor but this had no benefit. After trying two different homoeopathic medicines for the symptoms of vaginal burning after sex Nathalie's homoeopath tried a new remedy. He made a medicine from Nathalie's partner's ejaculate which, given in the 12c potency, allayed the irritation, and she was soon pregnant. The same medicine, given the name Seman hominum, was prescribed years later to a woman with an identical reaction. She became pregnant too. It is likely that both these women were allergic to some component of their partner's ejaculate.

17

Massage and Aromatherapy

There are various forms of massage, and while massage will not directly change a subfertile state to a fertile state, it has been included here as many practitioners use it as an adjunct to their main treatment – to relieve stress and tension and stimulate and tone internal organs.

Swedish massage, often called the 'gentle' massage, incorporates several types of movement to effect both relaxation and stimulation. It works on the soft tissue of the body – the muscles, vascular, lymphatic and nervous systems, through reflex action. While it has never been shown to have a direct benefit on fertility enhancement, you will know if you have experienced the luxury of massage just how relaxed and good you feel from a treatment. Swedish massage is used in aromatherapy treatments to aid oil penetration, and many practitioners combine the essential oils with their treatments.

Reiki is another gentle form of 'hands on' therapy which balances and promotes the healing on physical, emotional and spiritual levels. It can be used with any other form of treatment.

Deep tissue massage techniques include *shiatsu* (from the Japanese *shi*, finger, and *atsu*, pressure), and *Chinese acupressure*, both of which are branches of oriental medicine which apply treatment to and affect the energy flow of the channels or meridians. It can be quite painful on occasions but the practitioner will always work within a patient's tolerance, and most often the experience can be termed 'a comforting pain'. In a full body massage, the flow follows the meridians; however, a treatment may use just a few specific points, generally between four and ten. Treatment is applied usually by fingers or thumbs but elbows can also be used.

Neuromuscular massage is another form of deep tissue massage developed by osteopaths, and executed by applying specific pressure by fingers and thumbs to influence nerves and other connective tissue such as ligaments and tendons. Again this can be painful, but the practitioner will modify his or her touch and the duration of the massage movement to work within the patient's tolerance level.

While your partner or a friend can give you a gentle massage, deep tissue massage must only be given by qualified practitioners.

Aromatherapy is another adjunctive therapy that many women like to use. Therapeutic oils are administered through inhalations and baths, but mainly through massage during which the oils are absorbed through the skin into the body fluids. The physiological actions can be via the nervous system and probably the endocrine system and provide a hormone-regulating effect. Massage carries the oils to the organs they have a specific affinity with. Massage also stimulates the circulation and enhances the elimination of toxic substances.

The oils are usually diluted and used in combination to promote healing on three levels: physical, mental, and emotional. It is thought that the main effects of aromatherapy on fertility are through mental and emotional relaxation. They are harvested from flowers, trees, leaves, fruit (pith), bark, and roots and contain many different chemical constituents – as do herbs – each with its own unique healing properties and fragrance. The oils are super-concentrated; just the smallest dose taken orally could be fatal. However, some medical doctors are accredited to prescribe orally.

These gorgeously perfumed oils can be strong medicine! Even if you wish to use the oils in conjunction with a home massage, this should be done with guidance, especially if you are trying to conceive. Some oils may stimulate menstrual bleeding, and may even cause a miscarriage, while other oils must be avoided during pregnancy.

Oils to avoid during pregnancy Calamus, basil, hyssop, marjoram, myrrh, pennyroyal, sage, thyme, wintergreen.

Aromatherapy can be used in conjunction with other treatments to enhance fertility when massages are usually carried out at specific times during your cycle.

18

Counselling

Counselling for sexual dysfunction is a specialized branch of psychotherapy, practised by only a few specialists. When no organic cause can be found for a dysfunctional problem, a couple may be referred to a sex therapist by their health professional. The therapist usually likes to see both partners, at least initially, despite the fact that many people seeking help consider the problem is theirs alone and nothing to do with the other partner. It is also important throughout the therapy for the couple to work together.

During your first appointment with a sex therapist you should be assessing them just as much as they are assessing you. A good relaxed rapport with your practitioner is most important in sex therapy. During the first appointment the therapist explains how he or she will work, and what is required from those seeking help. The most important question the therapist will have in this regard is 'Do you have time to work at this problem at home?' The hourly sessions are all talking.

Initially, a thorough case history is taken for both parties, for sometimes the sexual aspect may be an expression of some other problem. All presenting issues are addressed and must be cleared for the treatment to be successful. Throughout the programme both parties work with the therapist.

Occasionally, a problem can be sorted out within the first consultation, but generally the therapy will consist of five to eight sessions. Because there is no formal training for sex therapists, each therapist develops their own way of working. The above represents one therapist's style. A qualified therapist has been properly trained, and you can contact the BAP to find a therapist in your area. (See the list of Useful Addresses at the back of the book.)

Greta and Peter's story

Greta and Peter had been married for 12 years and described their early relationship as 'passionate'. They had built up a successful business together, and after working all day made sure they had time to be with their two children aged six and four. After their second child, their sex life had gone steadily downhill. For the past four months Greta's libido had been non-existent. Peter felt resentful and rejected. They did not want to go to a counsellor and thought they should be able to resolve their problem alone. Counselling revealed power struggles and resentments that had built up over the years, but highlighted a basically strong marriage and two people who loved each other enough to want to make changes.

The sessions helped them appreciate how little time they had been spending together, just for themselves. They made a deliberate effort to change their routine and find time for each other. For them sex therapy was a successful and rewarding experience.

Ellen's story

Ellen suffered from vaginismus (severe vaginal pain which prevented intercourse). She had spent all her life on a farm, and when she married it was to a farmer. All her friends were having babies, and part of Ellen wanted a baby too. But another part of her was terrified. She would not go to a doctor as she feared an examination. It was not until the third session she very quietly asked her counsellor how far up the doctor would put his hand and arm inside her (thinking of the vet with the animals on the farm). She had no knowledge of the way her body worked or how it was put together. So with her husband, they worked through her fears, which then allowed her to go on and resolve the physical side of the problem through the approved protocol for vaginismus. And Ellen did have her baby, with very little fear at all.

Recommended Reading

The Fertility Awareness Workbook,
Barbara Kass-Annese & Dr Hal Danzer,
Hunter House, 1992

Getting Pregnant,
Prof. Robert Winston,
Pan, 1993

Natural Fertility,
Francesca Naish,
Milner, 2000

Overcoming Fertility: A Compassionate Resource to Getting Pregnant,
Prof. Robert Jansen,
W.H. Freeman, 1997

Preparation for Pregnancy: An essential guide,
Suzanne Gail Bradley & Nicholas Bennett,
Argyll, 1997

Sexual Chemistry,
Dr Ellen Grant,
Mandarin, 1996

Nutrition

Fats That Heal, Fats That Kill,
Udo Erasmus,
Alive Books, 1996

The New Nutrition,
Dr Michael Colgan,
CI Publications, 1994

Traditional Foods Are Your Best Medicine,
Roland F. Schmid,
Healing Arts Press, 1997

Western Diseases: Their emergence and prevention,
D. Burkitt & H. Trowell,
Harvard University Press, 1981

The Environment

'The Adverse Effects of Food Additives on Health',
Tuula E. Tuormaa,
Journal of Orthomolecular Medicine 9: 4, 1994.
Reprinted for Foresight.

'Adverse Effects of Agrochemicals on Reproduction and Health',
Tuula E. Tuormaa,
Journal of Nutrition & Environmental Medicine 5: 353–366, 1995.
Available as a review paper from Foresight.

Our Stolen Future,
T. Colborn, D. Dumanoski & J. Peterson-Myers,
Abacus, 1997

Perils of Progress,
John Ashton & Ron Laura,
Zed Books, 1999

Rachel's Environment & Health Weekly No. 599,
Environmental Research Foundation,
erf@rachel.org

Botanical (Herbal Medicine)

The Dictionary of Modern Herbalism,
Simon Mills,
MJF Books, 1997

Aromatherapy

The Art of Aromatherapy,
Robert Tisserand,
CW Daniel Co Ltd, 1992

Useful Addresses

Acupuncturists

British Acupuncture Council
63 Jeddo Road
London
W12 9HQ
Tel. 020 8735 0400

Homoeopaths

Homeopathic Medical Association
6 Livingstone Road
Gravesend
Kent
DA12 5DZ
Tel. 01471 560 336

Society of Homeopaths
4a Artizan Road
Northampton
NN1 4HU
Tel. 01604 621 400

Naturopaths

Association of Holistic Therapists
Flat 8
Soar Court
Scoff Street
Tenewydd
Rhondda
CR42 5NA
Tel. 01442 771 804

Osteopaths

Osteopathy Information Service
Osteopathy House
176 Tower Bridge Road
London
SE1 3LU
Tel. 020 7357 6655

Aromatherapy

Aromatherapy Organisations Council
3 Latymer Close
Braybrooke
Market Harborough
LE16 8LN
Tel. 01858 434 242

Personal Education

British Association of Psychotherapists
37 Mapesbury Road
London
NW2 4HJ
Tel. 020 8452 9823

Support/Advice

Family Planning Association
2–12 Pentonville Road
London
N1 9FP
Tel. 020 7837 5432

Fertility UK
Clitherow House
1 Blythe Mews
Blythe Road
London
W14 0NW
Tel. 020 7371 1341

Foresight
The Association for the Promotion of Pre-Conceptual Care
28 The Paddock
Godalming
Surrey
GU7 1XD
Tel. 01483 427 839

Environmental Research Foundation
PO Box 5036
Annapolis
MD 21403
USA

Index